T0008703

Romanticize Your Life

365 Simple Ways to Embrace the Beauty of Every Day

Jordan Ackerman

Illustrated by Amber Day

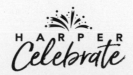

HARPER
Celebrate

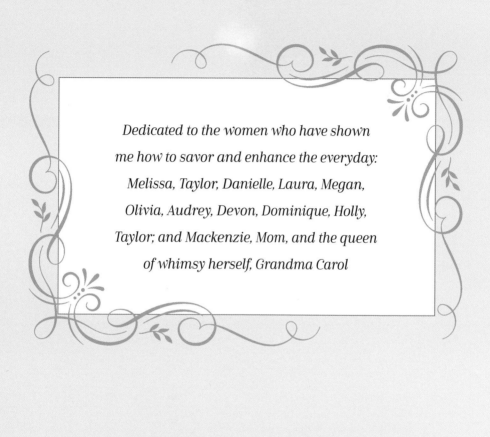

*Dedicated to the women who have shown
me how to savor and enhance the everyday:
Melissa, Taylor, Danielle, Laura, Megan,
Olivia, Audrey, Devon, Dominique, Holly,
Taylor; and Mackenzie, Mom, and the queen
of whimsy herself, Grandma Carol*

Romanticize Your Life

Copyright © 2023 Harper Celebrate

All rights reserved. No portion of this book may be reproduced, stored in a retrieval system, or transmitted in any form or by any means—electronic, mechanical, photocopy, recording, scanning, or other—except for brief quotations in critical reviews or articles, without the prior written permission of the publisher.

Published by Harper Celebrate, an imprint of HarperCollins Focus LLC.

Text by Jordan Ackerman.

Cover art and illustrations by Amber Day.

Any internet addresses (websites, blogs, etc.) in this book are offered as a resource. They are not intended in any way to be or imply an endorsement by HarperCollins Focus LLC, nor does HarperCollins Focus LLC vouch for the content of these sites for the life of this book.

ISBN 978-1-4002-4346-4 (epub)
ISBN 978-1-4002-4345-7 (HC)

Printed in Malaysia

23 24 25 26 27 OFF 5 4 3 2 1

Contents

To romanticize the world is to make us aware
of the magic, mystery and wonder of the world;
it is to educate the senses to see the ordinary
as extraordinary, the familiar as strange, the
mundane as sacred, the finite as infinite.

NOVALIS, German aristocrat, poet, author, mystic,
and philosopher of early German Romanticism

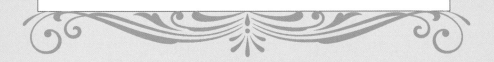

A Letter to Readers

Please read while narrating in the voice of the beloved Julie Andrews.

Dearest reader,

It's time to romanticize your life.

In an ever-changing world and a culture that often places value on speed and efficiency over experience, there is a deep need for us to slow down and savor the unique magic found in ordinary days.

Through every high and low, every big event and fleeting moment, exists the beauty and sacredness of your one unique life—and that is a gift worth celebrating. There is both satiating contentment and extraordinary wonder to be found in the smallest of moments in your days.

Here's the secret: the decadence is in the details of the life you're already living.

A satisfying life is often found in the minutiae, the all-too-often missed moments of sweetness in everyday occurrences. There are small, simple ways to approach these forgotten opportunities with the kind of curiosity and intentionality that create an internal joy that radiates outward.

Over the next 365 days, you'll explore a multitude of original ways to find inspiration for creativity, community, and self-care. Each month you'll also revisit recurring themes that will help you establish efficient routines, mindsets, and emotional reflections that will create a solid foundation so you can free yourself from stress and comparison to embrace your life more fully. By adopting a childlike wonder, intentional presence, and viewing your experiences through a lens of gratitude, you can begin romanticizing your life—starting today.

Theme Index

To serve as a guide, this index of key words will help you focus on various aspects of romanticizing your life. You'll see these listed in each entry.

———✥———

Consider the following as you experience this book:

Delight in the loveliness of ordinary days | Beauty

Recapture the magic of childhood | Whimsy

Listen to your needs and fill your emotional cup | Self-Care

Strengthen relationships and community | Connect

Invigorate your creative energy | Create

Cultivate a nurturing environment for yourself and others | Home

Seek out newness and adventure | Experience

Find rejuvenation in the great outdoors | Nature

Replenish your energy with a bit of comfort | Coziness

Celebrate who you are as a main character | Identity

Imagine all the dreams your heart desires | Dream

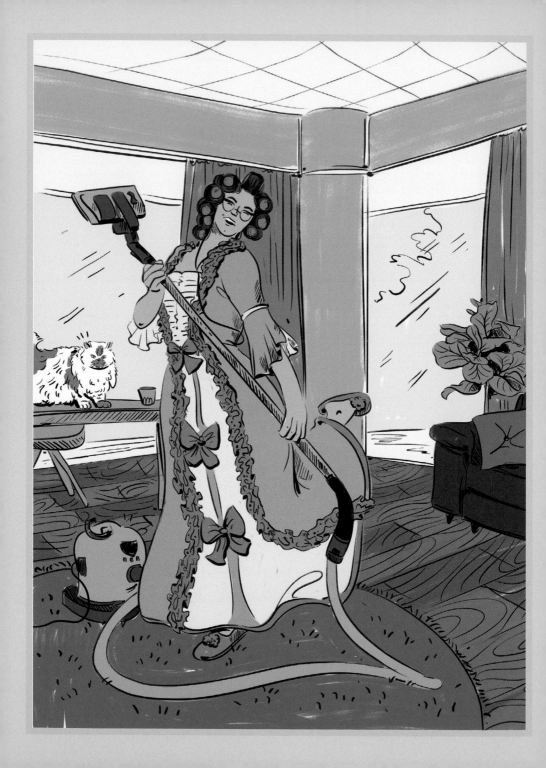

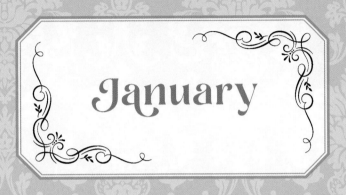

January

JANUARY 1
Never Too Late
Identity, Dream, Whimsy

Screenwriter Eric Roth helps to start us off on our journey toward romanticizing our lives. No matter where you are in life, his is a good reminder.

For what it's worth: it's never too late or, in my case, too early to be whoever you want to be. There's no time limit, stop whenever you want. You can change or stay the same, there are no rules to this thing. We can make the best or the worst of it. I hope you make the best of it. And I hope you see things that startle you. I hope you feel things you never felt before. I hope you meet people with a different point of view. I hope you live a life you're proud of. If you find that you're not, I hope you have the courage to start all over again.

ERIC ROTH, *The Curious Case of Benjamin Button*

JANUARY 2

Dream a Little Dream

Dream, Create

> I don't know yet what it is, or where it will be in reality, but I
> have a little house o' dreams all furnished in my imagination.

L. M. MONTGOMERY, *Anne's House of Dreams*

Today you are going to give yourself the permission to dream—to let your heart lead wherever it may. Grab some magazines, print out posts you've saved on social media, and round up some glue and scissors. Begin collaging together a dream board of these images: things you love, things you hope for, places you'd like to go, or the person you'd like to become.

Today isn't about forcing, striving, or creating a five-year plan. It's just about gathering, observing, and delighting in these desires of your heart. It's about seeing what you truly want, without judgment or expectation.

JANUARY 3
Sit in the In-between
Nature

Every realm of nature is marvelous.

ARISTOTLE, *On the Parts of Animals*

Step outside today, bundled up against winter's chill, paying attention to the small details that often go unnoticed as you hurry from place to place: the glint of sun upon an icy pathway, that crunchy crackle of boots on dried ground, or the particular scent of winter-crisp air.

JANUARY 4
Find the Fun
Whimsy, Experience

The character Mary Poppins taught us to find the fun when there's work to be done. Think of a chore you often dread, and brainstorm ways to make it more enjoyable. Whether it's playing upbeat music, listening to a podcast, or treating yourself to a reward after the chore is complete, channel your inner Mary Poppins today.

JANUARY 5

Cozy Up

Self-Care, Coziness

Combat winter's frigid nights with a bit of coziness. As you wind down for the evening, toss a blanket or sheet in the dryer for a few minutes. (Of course, check the laundry care instructions to determine if it's dryer safe!) Once warmed, pull out your layers of coziness, and curl up with a good book, your journal, or your current go-to television show.

JANUARY 6

Create Your Hometown Field Guide

Create, Home

Create a map of where you live, marked with your favorite places: restaurants, parks, shops, landmarks, even your favorite neighborhood streets. Save this to use as your field guide when out-of-town friends come to visit.

JANUARY 7
Choose Your January Theme Song
Whimsy

Imagine for a moment that your life is a movie—and you, my friend, are the main character! What's your January theme song to kick-start the year? Blast it from the car speakers with the windows down and with the cool wind in your hair, or listen to it via headphones as you move from scene to scene throughout your day.

JANUARY 8
Home Sweet Home
Home

Create a list of words to describe how you want your home to feel. *Chic, cozy, traditional, modern, eclectic*? Don't overthink it; just let the words flow, and see what inspirations emerge. What elements of your personality can you see reflected in the tone you aim to create?

JANUARY 9
No Need to Rush Your Dream
Dream

> I was thirty-two when I started cooking; up until then,
> I just ate.
>
> JULIA CHILD, American cooking teacher,
> author, and TV personality

After a successful career in foreign services, Julia Child started studying cooking when her husband's position—also in foreign services—led them to Paris. Julia didn't seriously dive into cooking until her thirties, when she enrolled in Le Cordon Bleu, Paris's famous cooking school.[1] The world-famous cook is legendary proof that it's possible to be multi-passionate and successful in diverse endeavors—and that it's never too late to dive into a new interest.

If you're feeling stuck, stalled out, or unsure of your current path, no need to fear! Keep pursuing the opportunities in front of you, along with the passions and hobbies that intrigue you. You never know what will unfold in the years to come.

JANUARY 10

HELLO, LOVER

Logophile

Whimsy

The English language has a number of *-phile* terms that refer to a person with fondness for specific topics, experiences, or things. Tracing back to Greek roots, the word *phile* comes from the ancient Greek word *philos*, meaning "to love."[2]

The modern English *-phile* terms are less commonly known and can take a few tries to pronounce correctly but are fun descriptors to know! Who do you know that is a logophile?

Logophile: a person with a fondness for words

JANUARY 11

House Shoes

Coziness, Self-Care

Buy yourself a pair of slippers or fuzzy socks to keep your feet warm during these colder months. It's amazing what a game changer warm feet can be as you lounge, cook, and get chores done.

JANUARY 12

Winter Walk

Nature, Experience

While blustery winter days aren't quite as enticing as the warmth of other seasons, you can still bundle up and enjoy the outdoors! Whether you head to a park, city garden, or hiking trail, layer up and head outside. The movement and change of scenery will give you a much-needed energy boost.

JANUARY 13

Storybook Escape

Whimsy

Reread one of your favorite books from childhood just for fun. Whether you have your own copy or borrow one from the library, read it out loud to yourself, letting the words fully surround you, transporting you back to fond childhood memories.

JANUARY 14
Explore a Museum
Experience

Take a stroll through a local museum, or explore a digital tour of a museum online. Let it transport you to another world, place, or time. Allow the exhibits to bring your attention to topics you don't typically dwell on. Perhaps it's classical art, past historical events, or scientific deep dives.

Select one exhibit to ponder what story its creators are trying to tell. What feelings are they aiming to evoke in visitors—wonder, gratitude, a desire to take action? Take note of how visitors are engaged through different visual, auditory, or tactile learning styles. How might what you've learned in the exhibit influence your life going forward?

JANUARY 15

Wake-Up Call

Self-Care

A consistent morning routine sets the tone for your entire day and helps to cultivate habits that support your overall physical, mental, and emotional health. There are simple ways to improve your morning routine and romanticize those early hours.

While the optimal wake-up time varies depending on the person, experts recommend waking up at the same time every day in order to help reinforce your natural circadian rhythm.[3] Figure out what time works best for you (it should ideally allow for around eight hours of sleep), and set your alarm clock to that time every day.

Maybe even try setting the alarm for a little earlier than you would typically like to wake up and resisting the temptation to hit that snooze button. It may be tough to get out of bed on the first few days, but as you get used to this schedule, you might just find that those early hours—when the sun streams in through the window and chirping birds greet the day in song—are especially sweet.

JANUARY 16

Do Some Soul-Searching

Identity, Dream

Set aside time to do some honest journaling about the person you currently are and the person you want to become. What are your strengths, and where do you have room for self-improvement? What values currently guide your decisions, and what values do you want to cultivate in order to become the person you want to be? What's one behavioral change that you can enact to begin to bridge that gap?

JANUARY 17

Create a Mood-Boost Playlist

Create, Experience

Create a playlist of your top twenty mood-boosting songs. Play it loud!

JANUARY 18

Send a Surprise

Connect

Why wait for a special occasion to brighten someone's day? Perhaps a friend has been going through a difficult time or someone you know is approaching a big life transition. The surprise doesn't have to be over-the-top or expensive. The smallest of gestures is a simple reminder that you're thinking of them, which might be just the pick-me-up they need.

JANUARY 19

Seek Out Starlight

Nature, Beauty

One of the few perks of limited daylight hours is how much easier it is to see the stars against the pitch-black sky earlier in the evening. Bundle up and do some winter stargazing! If you want to stay protected from the cold, stargaze through the window of a local café or the window of your own home.

JANUARY 20

Celebrate the Lunar New Year

Experience

Traditionally celebrated in Southeast Asian cultures, Lunar New Year marks the first lunar cycle of the new calendar year. The Chinese zodiac associates each year with an animal, which is traditionally used to anticipate the themes and fortune that year will bring.

The specific date for the Lunar New Year varies, so look up what day it will be this year. Then find a local lantern celebration you can attend with friends—or host one in your own backyard!

JANUARY 21

Take What You Need

Whimsy, Self-Care

Take what you need, and carry it with you for the rest of your day:

- lightness to laugh at yourself
- commitment to work through something challenging
- space to reflect on how you are feeling
- confidence that you can adapt to the unexpected

JANUARY 22
Begin Cultivating Those Dreams
Dream

Dreams are lovely. But they are just dreams. Fleeting,
ephemeral, pretty. But dreams do not come true just because
you dream them. . . . It's hard work that creates change.

SHONDA RHIMES, television producer,
screenwriter, and author

Earlier this month you were prompted to create a dream board of things
you love, things you hope for, places you'd like to go, the person you'd
like to become. Step one was to just gather and observe those dreams.
Now that you've had some time to sit with them, it's time for phase two:
intentional planning, research, and consistent effort.

Pick one hope, dream, or goal you would like to accomplish this year.
Are there any big milestones you'll need to hit to make it happen? Any
dependencies that will make or break it? Jot down your notes in your
journal or planner, and start cultivating!

While things likely won't go *exactly* as planned, breaking down your
dreams into their smaller components will help you get one step closer
each day to the life you are craving.

JANUARY 23
Candy Decor
Home, Create

Buy a bag of colorful candies and put them in a clear jar or pretty dish on display in your home.

JANUARY 24
Life Energy List
Self-Care, Identity

Create a list of the things that energize you, brighten your day, and spark joy. Keep adding to this list as things come to mind in the days ahead. This practice will give you a foolproof guide to turn to when you're in need of a pick-me-up.

JANUARY 25
Pretend to Be Psyched
Self-Care, Identity

Sometimes you just have to put on lip gloss and pretend to be psyched.

MINDY KALING, *Is Everyone Hanging Out Without Me? (And Other Concerns)*

Everyone has those days that they are less than psyched to have to show up for. The trick is to find the thing that will lift your spirits so you can take an energizing breath and say, "Let's do this."

Whether it's putting on lip gloss, wearing an outfit that makes you feel like a million bucks, or listening to a pump-up song before walking out the door, find your prep cue that will help you dive into the day with the mindset you need to set you up for success.

JANUARY 26
Savor Life's Little Fractions
Whimsy

The happiness of life . . . is made up of minute fractions—
the little, soon-forgotten charities of a kiss, a smile, a
kind look, a heartfelt compliment in the disguise of
playful raillery, and the countless other infinitesimals
of pleasurable and genial feeling.

SAMUEL TAYLOR COLERIDGE, *The Improvisatore*

As you go about your day, where can you add just one percent more
kindness? One percent more playfulness? Maybe one more smile? One
more moment of stillness?

These little fractions and percentages and just-one-mores add up
to creating beautiful days—and beautiful days add up to cultivating a
beautiful life.

JANUARY 27

Foundational Needs

Self-Care

Main-character energy doesn't just apply to your career, style, and relationships; it also applies to your finances! That's right: *you* are in the driver's seat, and financial stability helps create the framework for a less stressful life.

Financial mastery begins with addressing your foundational needs, which include housing, utilities, food, transportation, and medical care.

If your finances are feeling a little unruly, a great first step toward gaining control is to experiment with finance-tracking systems to find the one that works best for you. Excellent budgeting apps can sync to your bank accounts, investments, and credit cards and help you track spending, bills, and long-term saving goals. Don't let the options intimidate you; just start experimenting, and see if you can find a system that fits your unique needs.

JANUARY 28
Diversify Your Menu
Create, Home

One cannot think well, love well, sleep well, if one
has not dined well.

VIRGINIA WOOLF, *A Room of One's Own*

Get out of that food rut. Dust off a cookbook, and make a recipe you've
never tried before, even if it sounds intimidating.

JANUARY 29
New Year, *Nouveau Toi*
Experience

Intrigued by a foreign language? If you crave being immersed in another
culture, there are several top-notch language learning apps (check out
Duolingo or Babbel), local foreign language meetups (check out groups
on Meetup), and in-person foreign language classes that can help you
build your skills.

C'est bon!

JANUARY 30
Cozy Up
Coziness, Self-Care

--- SWEDISH WORD OF THE DAY ---

Mysa: a concept of contentment and coziness, often found at home, when engaging in a comforting activity

JANUARY 31
JANUARY REFLECTIONS
Delight in the Loveliness of Ordinary Days
Beauty

When we think of life's anticipations, we often focus on the big things, such as rights of passage, hard-won achievements, and long-awaited vacations.

But what are the little things you're looking forward to this year? Spend some time reflecting on the small delights the past month has offered, and dream up how you can create more opportunities to cultivate beauty within your ordinary days in the year ahead.

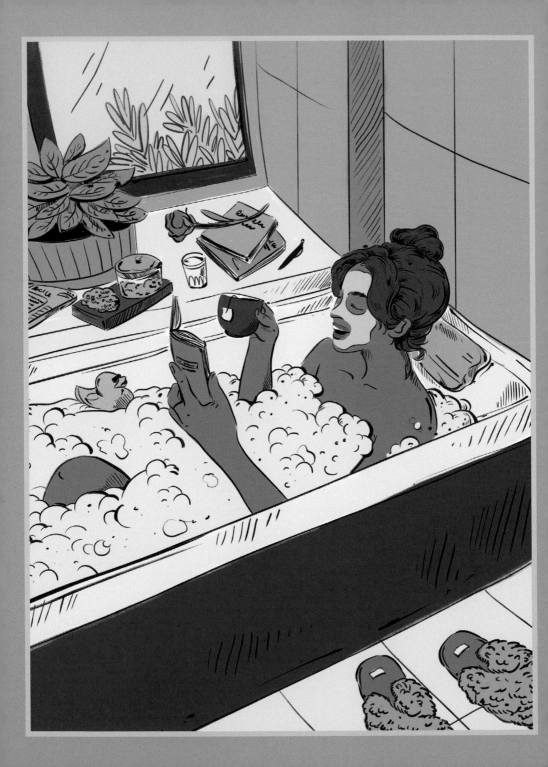

February

FEBRUARY 1
Seeing Clearly
Whimsy, Connect

It is only with one's heart that one can see clearly. What
is essential is invisible to the eye.

ANTOINE DE SAINT-EXUPÉRY, *The Little Prince*

What are the character traits you find most attractive, inspirational,
and admirable? Take five minutes to write these down. If you're feeling
stuck, think about the people in your life whom you admire and why.
Keep your eyes out this week for qualities you notice in those around
you, and add those to the list.

FEBRUARY 2
Give an Outfit a New Life
Create

Go thrifting for a new outfit! Head to a local resale shop, or check out
online clothing resale sites to give a previously owned outfit a new life.

FEBRUARY 3
Stand for Something
Identity, Self-Care

> Laugh as much as you choose, but you will not laugh me
> out of my opinion.
>
> JANE AUSTEN, *Pride and Prejudice*

What matters to you *really*? What stirs your soul or calls you to action? Determine the values, causes, or needs that most matter to you—and then look for ways to turn that passion into purpose.

FEBRUARY 4
Bring the Outside In
Home, Nature

Why not bring the outside in to get you through the rest of this chilly season? Head to a local plant shop to find a new piece of greenery to add to a happy little nook in your home. Plus, studies show their presence also boosts mood, creativity, and the ability to concentrate on the tasks at hand.[4]

FEBRUARY 5
Plan a Movie Date
Connect

Reach out to a friend and plan to catch a movie playing at a local theater. Better yet, grab an early showing so you can hang out and debrief on the movie afterward.

FEBRUARY 6
Teatime for All the Senses
Coziness, Self-Care

On a cold winter night, make yourself a steamy cup of bedtime tea. Pick your favorite non-caffeinated flavor.

As the kettle heats up, listen to the hum of the water warming and bubbles beginning to rise. After you pour your cup, curl up in a quiet spot in the house. Perhaps on the couch, by a fire, or looking out a window. Wrap your hands around the cup and feel its warmth. Breathe in the steam—watch it rise and swirl as it disappears. Enjoy the aromas as they release, creating the taste you so enjoy.

What a gift it is to be able to hear, to see, to feel, to smell, and to taste. Even the smallest moments are a gift.

FEBRUARY 7
Choose Your February Theme Song
Whimsy

What song will you play during your February montage?

Would a romantic ballad accompany you as you peruse the grocery store's flower selection of reds and pinks?

A song from the soundtrack of one of your favorite romantic movies?

Maybe a classic love song from the 1950s?

Or perhaps it's a string quartet that provides the background music as winter's chill is warmed by the impending spring?

Whatever the song may be, feel all the feels and fully embrace this month's mood. Let February's theme song fill you with music to encourage you during the process of romanticizing your life so that it becomes second nature.

FEBRUARY 8

ROMANTICISM LESSON

Romanticism's Roots

Whimsy

Believe it or not, the Romantic movement isn't a new one; it emerged in the late 1700s in northern Europe.

Here's a quick overview of Romanticism's roots, according to The Art Story Foundation:

At the end of the 18th century and well into the 19th, Romanticism quickly spread throughout Europe and the United States to challenge the rational ideal held so tightly during the Enlightenment. The artists emphasized that sense and emotions—not simply reason and order—were equally important means of understanding and experiencing the world. Romanticism celebrated the individual imagination and intuition in the enduring search for individual rights and liberty. Its ideals of the creative, subjective powers of the artist fueled avant-garde movements well into the 20th century.[5]

FEBRUARY 9
Decor Refresh
Home, Create

Remember that list you started back in January about how you want your home to feel? Now it's time to use it to refresh the decor in an area of your home that seems a bit stale.

Before heading to the store for new items, try shopping your own home! Hunt through closets, storage bins, and other rooms in your place to see what you can mine from what you already have on hand. Sometimes all it takes is a little rearranging to create a whole new feeling.

FEBRUARY 10
HELLO, LOVER
Clinophile
Whimsy

Clinophile: a lover of reclining, lounging, or lying in bed

Calling all loungers! How can you spruce up your favorite place to recline? Perhaps a new decorative pillow? A cozy throw?

FEBRUARY 11
Enjoy a Seasoned Cauliflower Steak
Create

Part of a well-lived life is prioritizing eating nourishing foods that make you feel great. Thankfully, you don't have to compromise flavor for nutrition—you can have both! These cauliflower steaks are a flavorful and nutrient-rich dish you can add to your dinner.

Seasoned Cauliflower Steaks
Prep time: 10 minutes | Cook time: 30 minutes | Serves: 3

Ingredients
2 medium heads of cauliflower

Olive oil spray

1 teaspoon kosher salt, divided

$1/2$ teaspoon black pepper, divided

1 teaspoon garlic powder, divided

1 teaspoon paprika, divided

1 teaspoon coriander, divided

Instructions

1. Preheat the oven to 425 degrees Fahrenheit. Line a large, rimmed baking sheet with foil or parchment paper, and spray it with olive oil.

2. Wash the cauliflower heads, then remove the outer leaves and trim the very bottom of the core but keep the core intact. Slice each head into 3/4-inch-thick slices. The outer slices will fall apart; you can simply roast them as florets along with the steaks. Each cauliflower head should yield three steaks.

3. Arrange the steaks in a single layer on the baking sheet. Scatter the florets around them. Spray their tops with olive oil, and sprinkle them with half the seasonings.

4. Bake the cauliflower pieces for 15 minutes.

5. Remove the cauliflower from the oven, then carefully flip the pieces, spray with more oil, and sprinkle with the remaining spices. Continue baking until browned and fork-tender, about 10 to 15 more minutes.

FEBRUARY 12
Define *Elegance*
Beauty, Identity

We must never confuse elegance with snobbery.

YVES SAINT LAURENT, French fashion designer
and cofounder of YSL fashion house

Take a few moments to define what *elegance* means to you. What does it look like when no one is watching? How does it shape the way you interact with others? What does it feel like to embody? Keep this in mind as you move throughout your day, and see if it impacts the way you feel about yourself and how that affects the way you present yourself to the world.

FEBRUARY 13
Work It
Experience

Try out a new exercise class! Whether it's a new studio for a workout you already love or a whole new form of movement, do something good for your body today.

FEBRUARY 14
Little Love Notes
Connect, Create

While Valentine's Day is often associated with commercialized cards and overpriced gifts, there is no better way to mark this holiday than by taking the opportunity to tell the people you love how very much they mean to you. Instead of spending money on generic store-bought cards, take a few minutes to handwrite notes to the most important people in your life, and pop them in the mailbox. This sweet, simple offering will make others feel so very loved.

FEBRUARY 15
RECALIBRATE YOUR MORNING ROUTINE
Make Your Bed
Self-Care, Beauty, Coziness

Starting your morning with this small step not only kicks off your day with intention and a clean, orderly slate, but it can also give you a little boost of satisfaction for having accomplished a task before you ever walk out the door. Revel in this daily tidy as you smooth out your bed linens, knowing that you're creating a welcoming place to rest in the evening to come.

FEBRUARY 16
Pinpoint Your Travel Aspirations
Dream

A great way to offset feelings of stagnant complacency is to dream up a list of places you would love to travel. Start by listing the places you've always wanted to go, then peruse some travel blogs to see if you discover any new destinations that spark your interest.

FEBRUARY 17
Host a Favorite Things Swap
Connect

Who doesn't love to share what they love? It's the perfect reason to host a "favorite things" party. Have each guest bring one of their current favorite things, all wrapped up. It could be a book they recently read, home product they are loving, favorite snack—you get the idea! As guests arrive, have them draw numbers from a hat to determine the order of gift selection. As gifts are opened, you can allow for a limited number of trades, or have everyone stick with the first present they pick. The most important part is that when a gift is opened, the person who brought it shares why it's one of their favorite things. What better way to spread joy this season?

FEBRUARY 18
Watch an Eye-Opening Documentary
Dream

There are many ways to become a lifelong learner. Instead of settling in to watch an episode of a scripted show this evening, search for a documentary about a topic that intrigues you. Maybe it's about something that has long piqued your interest, or maybe it's about a subject you've never even pondered before. Let yourself get pulled into the story, and delight in expanding your mind beyond your everyday.

FEBRUARY 19
Beauty Begins
Beauty, Identity

Beauty begins the moment you decide to be yourself.

COCO CHANEL (ATTRIBUTED)

Today, make a list of the top ten things you find beautiful about yourself—inside and out.

FEBRUARY 20
Tend to the Hands That Tend to Life's Needs
Self-Care

Your hands work hard, and the winter months are especially harsh on your skin. Today, tend to the hands that tend to all of your life's needs. Head to a salon, or pick up polish and supplies for an at-home manicure. Maybe try a new, nourishing hand cream. If there's someone in your life who works extra hard to take care of others, invite that person along so they can feel taken care of for a change.

FEBRUARY 21
Take What You Need
Whimsy, Self-Care

Take what you need, and carry it with you for the rest of your day:

- belief that you are enough
- strength to push through obstacles
- energy to finish something you've started
- satisfaction with a job well done

FEBRUARY 22
Let Beautiful Things Find You
Beauty, Whimsy

As you're going through your day today, be on the lookout for all things beautiful. Perhaps you're having the type of day that requires added effort, but just take a moment and look—maybe look outside of a window, or maybe up at the sky. Maybe do an internet search on beautiful flowers or trees or faces. Maybe the way someone offered you your coffee came with a beautiful smile. If you're not already present to the abundance of beauty in the world, how might you let beauty find you today?

FEBRUARY 23
Dance the Night Away
Experience

Want to step into another decade, another place, or another culture? So often we view food as the go-to vehicle to transport ourselves, but why not learn a dance? Whether it's the waltz, salsa, Kathak, or even the choreography from your favorite throwback music video, take the opportunity to step outside your comfort zone and learn a dance just for fun!

FEBRUARY 24
Set the Mood
Home, Experience

Dim the lights, light some candles, and turn on a jazzy cooking playlist while you make dinner.

FEBRUARY 25
Start Planning Your Voyage
Dream

Remember last week when you jotted down your dream travel list? Today, pick one location and start gathering some itinerary ideas. Look up travel guides on Pinterest, location-based social media accounts, or travel blogs. Use these as a springboard to create your customized travel plan!

FEBRUARY 26
Curate Your Thoughts
Self-Care

Watch your thoughts, they become words;

watch your words, they become actions;

watch your actions, they become habits;

watch your habits, they become character;

watch your character, it becomes destiny.

FRANK OUTLAW (ATTRIBUTED)

These wise words can truly help to cultivate the type of life you live, romanticized or not. As you go about today—and the next day, and the next—become intentional about your thoughts. For example, think on lovely and beautiful things and you will speak of lovely and beautiful things— which contribute to creating a life full of loveliness and beauty.

FEBRUARY 27
Remember the Difficulty in Learning
Whimsy, Identity

All things are difficult, before they are easy.

THOMAS FULLER, *Gnomologia*

All of the great thinkers, philosophers, and teachers started somewhere. Being a beginner is deceptively exhausting. Nothing is second nature; everything must be done with full attention and analysis. Whether it's writing a press release, using a new technology at work, or organizing a social event, with newness comes difficulty.

In what areas of life are you a beginner right now? Extend yourself grace for the challenges and energy expenditure that will naturally accompany these tasks until you gain more experience, and trust that they will indeed become easier with time.

FEBRUARY 28

Recapture the Magic of Childhood

Whimsy

Give yourself the gift of looking through a child's eyes today. Imagine, just for a moment, that you know not of the world's weary ways. Reflect on some of the things you used to love doing when you were very young.

Getting lost in the fictional world of a book or movie? Creating imaginary adventures starring the clouds' shapes in the blue sky above? Maybe just allowing yourself the space to sit still and do absolutely nothing?

Delight in that innocence; revel in that hope. How can you hold on to this sense of whimsy in the days ahead?

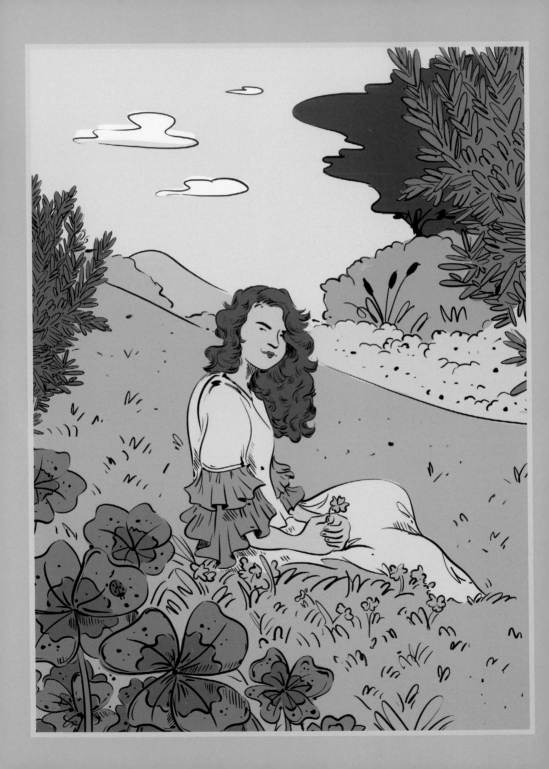

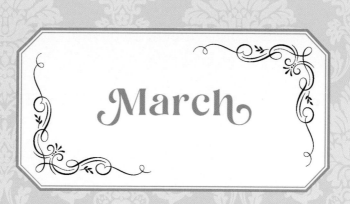

March

MARCH 1

Cultivate Connection to Combat Dread

Dream, Experience, Connect

All we have to decide is what to do with the time that is
given us.

J.R.R. TOLKIEN, *The Fellowship of the Ring*

Think of somewhere you go routinely that you've started to . . . well . . .
kind of dread. It could be the grocery store, a weekly work meeting, or
the bus stop for your daily commute. How could you mix things up,
changing the atmosphere in that space and facilitating connections
with the people there?

Could you blast the Beach Boys when sitting in the school pickup
line? Strike up conversation with the grocery cashier? Bake a fun treat
to liven up your team meetings at work?

Rather than let dread keep you down, take a simple step to cultivate
a more uplifting atmosphere in those routine spaces. Your small effort
might just be the big spark you needed.

MARCH 2

Homemade Face Mask

Self-Care

Take care of yourself every day as a matter of course,
as you would dress or undress; and be sure that health
is coming. Say over and over to yourself: Nourishment,
fresh air, exercise, rest, patience.

ANNIE PAYSON CALL

Time to pamper yourself—starting in your own kitchen! You'd be surprised what coffee grounds, sugar, or that jar of honey can be transformed into. Look up a homemade facial-scrub recipe online that uses ingredients you have on hand, and pamper away!

MARCH 3

Think Beautifully

Beauty, Whimsy

——————— GREEK WORD OF THE DAY ———————

Eunoia: a pure and well-balanced mind that shows kindness and goodwill to others; beautiful thinking

MARCH 4

Springtime Essentials

Identity

As the seasons change, so do your needs. Create a list of your springtime essentials. This includes playlists, style items, activities, places, and the must-haves floating around in your purse.

MARCH 5

Savor the Moments

Whimsy, Experience, Self-Care

We do not remember days, we remember moments.…
The richness of life lies in memories we have forgotten.

CESARE PAVESE

Start keeping a moments journal. Each evening list three moments you're grateful for or want to remember from that day. This practice will shape the story you're telling yourself as you close each day and will help your mind tune in to those special micro-moments that you'll want to carry with you forever.

MARCH 6

Magazine Date

Self-Care

Remember your days as a teenager when you'd spend ages flipping through magazines? How about reliving those fond memories just for a couple of hours? Head to a local grocery store or bookstore, and browse away! Choose your favorite magazine to purchase, then head to a cute coffee shop or café to flip through the pages uninterrupted—a blissful reprieve from all the tasks on your to-do list.

MARCH 7

Choose Your March Theme Song

Whimsy

Spring has sprung! Birds are chirping, flowers are in bloom, and the air is crisp with the changing of seasons and new possibilities. Choose a March theme song that encapsulates the feeling of the warm spring sun breaking through the clouds of winter.

MARCH 8
Broaden Your Circle
Experience

If you're feeling stir-crazy, stagnant, or just a bit blah, carve out ten minutes to look up *Time* magazine's the TIME 100, its annual list of the one hundred most influential people in the world. Every year *Time* identifies one hundred people across the globe who are having the greatest impact on art, culture, politics, and humanitarian well-being.

Your eyes will be opened to amazing men and women, many whose names you've never even heard before. See whose stories spark your interest, broaden your empathy, or grow your awareness of wonders being done around the world.

MARCH 9
Closet Clean-Out
Home, Experience

Take a look through your closet, and see what pieces aren't speaking to you in the way they used to. Donate gently used items to a local charity, and let someone else give them a renewed life.

MARCH 10
Talk, Write, or Cry It Out
Self-Care

A mermaid has no tears, and therefore she suffers so much more.

HANS CHRISTIAN ANDERSEN, *The Little Mermaid*

While positivity, perseverance, and a can-do attitude are all wonderful qualities, if you've been pushing away your less-than-bubbly feelings for a while now, you're likely long overdue for a venting session with a trusted friend, a quiet window for some raw journaling, or even a good cry.

Studies show that acknowledging, naming, and feeling our emotions (yes, especially the harder, heavier ones) is crucial for our mental and physical well-being.[6] Experiencing these feelings allows our brains to process them, decreasing their intensity and shortening the time they negatively impact us.

MARCH 11

Managing Loans

Self-Care

> But what madness it must be to run in debt for these superfluities?

BENJAMIN FRANKLIN

Debt is often an inevitable part of life. Whether you take out a loan to finance your education, a car, a home, a new business, it's a tool that sets you up for success down the road, but it can create stress while the debt looms overhead.

It's important to check in to make sure you're staying on track with paying off student debt, loans, and credit cards, if any of those apply to you. If interest rates have gone down, look into refinancing the loan. Or, while evaluating your income, see if it makes sense to start putting more money down to pay off the loan more quickly. You are capable of managing this, one small step at a time.

MARCH 12
Casting Call
Dream, Identity

Time for your very own casting call! If a movie was made about your life, what actor would you want to play you? What character traits of yours would be most important for that actor to embody? What actors would you want to play your friends and family? Share your choices with them, and see if they agree.

MARCH 13
Host a Book Club
Connect

Rally a group of friends to read a book and then meet up to discuss it. You could select a book that opens your eyes to perspectives you aren't exposed to every day, a title that cultivates self-reflection, or a suspenseful thriller that keeps you guessing at the turn of every page.

Whatever genre you decide on, have everyone come to your book chat with a discussion topic or a question the book sparked for them. This will get the conversation going and give everyone a chance to share a bit about how the book affected them.

MARCH 14
Add a Lucky Charm
Create

Find a new bauble to add to your key ring. While it may not be a true lucky charm, it will add some fun to your everyday.

MARCH 15
RECALIBRATE YOUR MORNING ROUTINE
Create a No-Phone Zone
Self-Care

Your brain produces five kinds of brain waves that operate at different speeds.[7] When you first wake up in the morning and you're in that daydreamy place between resting and wakefulness, your brain is in an ideal state for the free flow of ideas and creativity. Reaching for your phone snaps you out of this realm and catapults you into the distractions of the outside world.

Instead of immediately turning to the screen, try starting your morning with quieter activities that will work with the rhythms of your brain activity instead of against them.

MARCH 16
Love's Only Remedy
Connect

There is no remedy for love but to love more.

HENRY DAVID THOREAU, *Journal 1: 1837–1844*

Where can you add a little more love in your life today?

Where can you express a little more love or loving-kindness to the people in your life?

For an extra challenge, see if you can be extra loving or kind today and this week to as many groups as you can in this list below:

close family members

extended family members

romantic partners

close friends

friends you haven't spoken with in a while

neighbors

coworkers—including your boss

service people

store clerks

government employees

MARCH 17
Meditate on the Words of Saint Patrick
Whimsy

Originating in Ireland, Saint Patrick's Day is a holiday filled with religious services, feasts, and celebrations in honor of the country's patron saint, Saint Patrick.

Below are a few verses from a prayer for protection frequently attributed to Saint Patrick, referred to as "Saint Patrick's Breastplate." Read these words aloud, and see what thoughts and feelings they stir within you.

> I arise today, through
> The strength of heaven,
> The light of the sun,
> The radiance of the moon,
> The splendor of fire,
> The speed of lightning,
> The swiftness of wind,
> The depth of the sea,
> The stability of the earth,
> The firmness of rock.

MARCH 18

International Vibes

Home

Turn on a vibey international playlist to change the atmosphere of your home. If you're feeling stumped, try French, Portuguese, Indian, Korean, or Chinese.

MARCH 19

Take a Meditative Bubble Break

Whimsy, Self-Care

Next time you're at the store, buy yourself a bottle of bubbles. When you need a moment to reset, head outside and relax into the childlike wonder that those captivating floating spheres of shimmering color sparked in you once upon a time. As you watch them pop, name each one with a positive word: *wonder*, *joy*, *happiness*, *love*, and so on.

MARCH 20
Springtime Affirmations
Self-Care, Identity

The words we speak over ourselves have power. They shape the lenses through which we view our experiences, as well as what we pay attention to, and ultimately the person we become.

What are some words you want to speak over yourself during this spring season? Think about how you typically feel during this time of year—physically, mentally, and emotionally—and jot down affirmations, prayers, or hopes for this season. Post the list somewhere you will see it daily. Reading these every day will surely have an impact!

MARCH 21
Let There Be Light
Home

The simple addition of an accent lamp in an unexpected spot can drastically change the look and feel of any area. Whether you're looking for a warm yellow glow to make your reading nook feel more cozy or a cool art deco lamp to add style to an otherwise bland space, a little lighting can really work wonders.

MARCH 22
Everyday Essentials
Whimsy

Every day . . . do something creative, something
generous, and something foolish.

These are the words of economist, professor, and investor Benjamin
Graham, according to one of his most famous mentees, Warren Buffett.
How can you intentionally accomplish each of these tasks today?

MARCH 23
Take What You Need
Whimsy, Self-Care

Take what you need, and carry it with you for the rest of your day:

- spaciousness
- boldness
- gentleness
- diligence

MARCH 24

Saving for Retirement

Self-Care

For age and want save while you may,
No morning sun lasts a whole day.

BENJAMIN FRANKLIN

While retirement may feel far away, investing early on in your future self makes a huge difference. Even small monthly investments will add up and grow! Set up your future self for financial success. Look into retirement planning through your place of work, or speak with a financial advisor to learn about your options.

Or read some of these classic books to help inspire and empower you in this area:

Rich Dad Poor Dad by Robert Kiyosaki
The Intelligent Investor by Benjamin Graham
The Way to Wealth by Benjamin Franklin
Think and Grow Rich by Napoleon Hill
The Total Money Makeover by Dave Ramsey

MARCH 25

Love

Whimsy

Part of Victorian-era etiquette included learning floriography, the symbolic language of flowers. Flowers were used to deliver messages that were not socially appropriate to be spoken aloud, as well as to reinforce thoughts and feelings that had been previously shared by the sender.[8]

Nearly all Victorian homes had, alongside the Bible, guidebooks for deciphering the "language," although definitions shifted depending on the source. Flowers could be used to express love, devotion, or romantic interest as well as hatred or conceit. How the flowers were delivered added another layer of messaging—with what hand they were delivered and on which side of the bouquet the ribbon was tied.

While the meanings and traditions have changed over time, the fascination with this gentle floral language persists just the same. Consider revitalizing this subtle language in your own life. Below is a list of just a few flowers that communicate sentiments of love:

> **red tulip**: passion, a declaration of love
>
> **sweet pea**: blissful pleasures, goodbye, "thank you for a lovely time"
>
> **gardenia**: secret love, "you're lovely"
>
> **pink carnation**: "I'll never forget you"
>
> **red rose**: love, "I love you"

MARCH 26

Establish Your Boundaries

Self-Care

> I want to protect each person's boundaries. Once you
> begin to yield the slightest ground on some pretext,
> you're ultimately left with nothing.

RABINDRANATH TAGORE

Today give yourself permission to:

- have boundaries and stick to them.
- be in a busy season and have less capacity for spontaneity.
- disappoint someone.

Boundaries can sometimes be tough to keep, but they are so important to your overall well-being. Don't be afraid to take the time and space you need.

MARCH 27

Learn About the Founders

Whimsy

Learn about Romanticism's roots by learning about the thought leaders who spearheaded the movement. Do some research on Ludwig Tieck, Karl Wilhelm Friedrich Schlegel, and August Wilhelm Schlegel. What did they believe, and how did those beliefs shape their work?

MARCH 28

Search for a Four-Leaf Clover

Whimsy, Nature

According to Irish tradition, those who find a four-leaf clover are destined for good luck. It is said that each of the four leaves symbolizes good omens for faith, hope, love, and luck.

Head outside and hunt for some good fortune today!

MARCH 29

That Certain Something

Whimsy

--- FRENCH PHRASE OF THE DAY ---

Je ne sais quoi: a quality or positive essence that cannot be easily described or expressed

MARCH 30

Pot a Shamrock Plant

Whimsy, Coziness

May your blessings outnumber the shamrocks that grow.
And may trouble avoid you wherever you go.

TRADITIONAL IRISH BLESSING

This is the time of year where you can find potted shamrocks from your local florist or grocer. Consider bringing one into your home to add some Irish cheer and set intentions for good luck to come your way.

MARCH 31

Fill Your Emotional Cup

Self-Care

You can't pour from an empty cup. As you reflect on the previous month, think about the ways in which you feel emotionally nourished. What fills you up and makes you feel as if you have more of yourself to give to others? Take the time to identify what helps you feel like the best version of you. Looking forward, how will you prioritize making time for this on a regular basis?

Let this excerpt from *Love, Life, & Work* by Elbert Hubbard inspire you:

The supreme prayer of my heart is not to be learned, rich, famous, powerful, or "good," but simply to be radiant. I desire to radiate health, cheerfulness, calm courage, and good will. I wish to live without hate, whim, jealousy, envy, fear. I wish to be simple, honest, frank, natural, clean in mind and clean in body, unaffected . . . ready to face any obstacle and meet every difficulty unabashed and unafraid. . . .

If I can help people, I'll do it by giving them a chance to help themselves; and if I can uplift or inspire, let it be by example, inference, and suggestion, rather than by injunction and dictation. That is to say, I desire to be radiant—to radiate life.

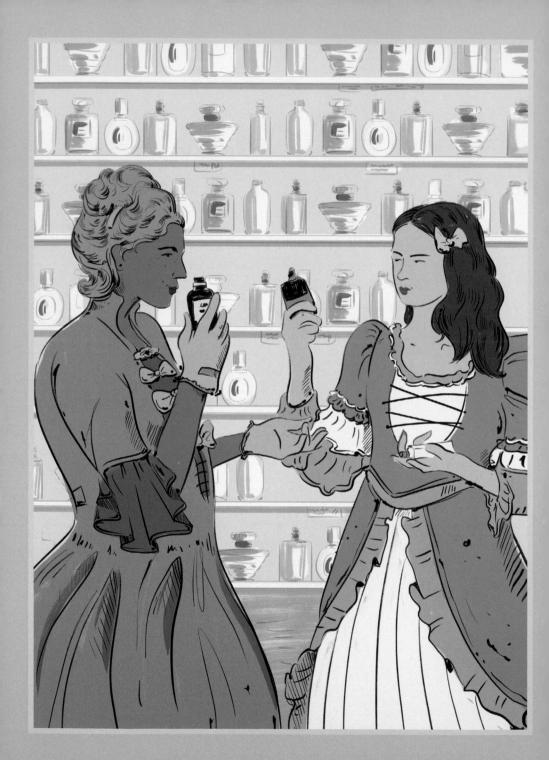

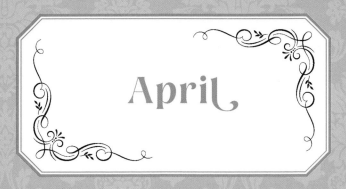

April

APRIL 1
Window Washing
Home

As terrible as this chore might sound, washing your windows will make your home feel like a radiant diamond once you're done. Set aside a block of time to wash your home's windows, inside and out. Removing that layer of dust, pollen, and grime will allow the spring sunlight in, and it might even brighten your outlook on life a little bit as well.

APRIL 2
Find Your Spring Scent
Beauty, Identity

Find your signature springtime scent! Whether it's perfume from a department store, a favorite combination of essential oils, or a candle to create a lovely ambience in your home, do some exploring to find a scent that feels like you in this season.

Freshness, happiness, and blooms are associated with this time of year, so search for scents with notes of bergamot, lemon, mandarin, and romantic florals like iris, jasmine, and rose.

APRIL 3

Highest Self

Identity

Visualize your highest self and start showing up as her. Write a list of qualities you want to embody. Post it somewhere you'll see it often, and begin to take mental stock of how you're aiming toward—and realizing—those valuable traits.

APRIL 4

Revamp Your Evening Routine

Self-Care

As spring begins to approach summer—with longer days and vacations—it can be easy to lose your grip on maintaining an evening routine that sets you up for success for the following day.

Take a thoughtful look at your evening routine. What can you add to your nightly task list that will help the next day run more smoothly? A quick five-minute house tidy? Tossing in a load of laundry? Slow stretches to get those kinks out of your muscles?

Brainstorm a simple evening routine that works for your most important needs.

APRIL 5
Lend a Hand
Connect, Identity

When you've worked hard, and done well, and walked
through that doorway of opportunity, you do not slam
it shut behind you. You reach back, and you give other
folks the same chances that helped you succeed.

MICHELLE OBAMA, From the 2012 Democratic
National Convention Speech[9]

Michelle Obama had a credentialed career before stepping into her
role as First Lady. A successful lawyer, community activist, nonprofit
founder, and hospital executive, Michelle learned the challenges of carving her path in the professional world, as well as the value of lending a
hand to those a step or two behind her.

Think about the ways others have helped you by sharing important lessons and connecting you with the people and resources you
needed to succeed. Now think about how you can do the same for others
behind you.

APRIL 6

Let Joy Take Flight

Connect, Nature, Experience, Whimsy

> The Kite is safe among the boughs; I can see its long tail
> hanging down. But do look here! The Kite has made us
> a present of five young rooks; two are fluttering among
> the golden pippins, and three are hopping and gaping
> among the gingerbread-nuts.
>
> HARRIET MYRTLE, *Adventure of a Kite*

Today feel the wind beneath your wings while keeping your feet on the ground.

On a day with a strong breeze, invite a friend or two to head to the store to purchase kites. (Yes, you read that correctly!)

Next, head to an open outdoor space—a park, a seashore, or an open field—and let joy take flight. Savor the first moment when the kite's wings catch the wind and the string pulls taut against your grip. Enjoy the dance between the wings and the wind, allowing the kite to keep climbing higher and higher and higher. There will be some inevitable crashes, which will make the moments of flight that much more glorious.

Who says only children can experience childlike joy?

APRIL 7

Choose Your April Theme Song

Whimsy

> April is the cruellest month, breeding
> Lilacs out of the dead land, mixing
> Memory and desire, stirring
> Dull roots with spring rain.
>
> T. S. ELIOT, "The Waste Land"

Pain and pleasure. Loss and gain. Sadness and joy.

As winter's frost melts and spring's new life grows, the month of April encapsulates the notion of feeling two things at once. Choose a theme song for this month that does the same.

APRIL 8

Make a Wildflower Bouquet

Experience, Nature, Beauty

Head out in search of wildflowers, and pick your very own bouquet of local blooms.

APRIL 9

Enjoy a Festival

Experience

Look up when local fairs and festivals will be taking place in your area this year, and mark your calendar with those that pique your interest so you'll be sure not to miss them!

APRIL 10

Choose Not to Be Harmed

Self-Care

> Choose not to be harmed—and you won't feel harmed.
> Don't feel harmed—and you haven't been.
>
> MARCUS AURELIUS, *Meditations: A New Translation*

You can't control the actions of others or many of life's challenging circumstances. You can control only how you respond. Are there any grievances you can let go of today? Try making the choice not to feel harmed by things you can't control.

APRIL 11
Embrace the Growing Pains
Dream, Identity

On these magic shores children at play are forever beaching their coracles. We too have been there; we can still hear the sound of the surf, though we shall land no more.

J. M. BARRIE, *Peter Pan*

Becoming the truest, fullest version of yourself means continuing to grow and evolve. It means trying things on and seeing how they fit— everything from relationships and hobbies to thought patterns and daily routines. While it's fun and exciting to cultivate the new parts of your life that truly feel right, it can feel uncomfortable and even sad to let go of the parts that are no longer aligned with the person you are becoming.

Jot down a list of habits, thought patterns, relationships, and ways you spend your time that have recently shifted or need to shift in order to allow you to keep growing. Express gratitude for the things you're leaving behind and how they served you, while also keeping your gaze fixed on the person you're becoming, the version of you that is fully thriving and living her best life.

APRIL 12

Freedom, Flowers, and Books

Whimsy, Nature

With freedom, flowers, books, and the moon,
who could not be perfectly happy?

OSCAR WILDE, *De Profundis*

APRIL 13

Create a Springtime Flat Lay

Create, Nature, Beauty

Head outside to your springtime pallet of buds, blooms, and new growth.
Gather flowers, foliage, and other natural materials, and arrange them
in an artistic flat lay—a fancy term for a visually appealing design from
a bird's-eye view—on the ground for passersby to enjoy.

APRIL 14
Garden Party
Connect, Experience

Host a lovely garden party—whether at your own home or a park. Offer bite-size eats and bubbly drinks, set up a croquet course or another lawn game, and put on your Sunday best. (If you want to go the extra mile, request that everyone speak in their best British accent!)

APRIL 15
RECALIBRATE YOUR MORNING ROUTINE
Face Time
Self-Care

Some dermatologists recommend washing your face in the morning with a gentle cleanser, while others say rinsing with water is enough, especially if you cleansed your face the evening before. (Over-cleansing could dry out your skin.) Determine what works best for your skin's unique needs, and delight in adding this simple pleasure to your morning routine. Imagine the water rinsing away the evening's hours and preparing your face to greet the day ahead.

APRIL 16

Open-Air Life

Whimsy, Nature

Friluftsliv: the concept of a simple life in nature, the valuable act of spending time in remote outdoor locations to enhance one's spiritual and physical well-being; literally translates to "open-air life"

APRIL 17

Savor Your Unique Loves

Connect, Coziness

There are all types of love in this world, but never the same love twice.

F. SCOTT FITZGERALD, "The Sensible Thing"

Think about how unique each relationship is in your life. We connect over different interests, special inside jokes, and memories that could never be replicated. Take a moment to note the relationships that you're most grateful for and some of the unique memories you share with each person.

APRIL 18
Two Helping Hands
Whimsy, Self-Care, Connect

Remember, if you ever need a helping hand, you'll find one at the end of your arm. As you grow older, you will discover that you have two hands: one for helping yourself, the other for helping others.

SAM LEVENSON, *In One Era and Out the Other*

Did you know that helping others can actually help yourself? According to an article titled "In Helping Others, You Help Yourself,"[10] published by *Psychology Today*, there's enough research to suggest that doing good deeds, both big and small, and helping others not only helps us to feel good but can also do some good for us physically.

Who in your life could you help out today?

What social causes tug on your heart and mind?

Where have you considered volunteering?

Take a leap and lend a helping hand, and maybe help romanticize someone else's life today.

APRIL 19

Reflect on April Showers

Self-Care

Sweet April showers,

Do spring May flowers.

THOMAS TUSSER, *Five Hundred Points of Good Husbandry*

A familiar phrase that captures a familiar rhythm of life—a season of dreariness or sadness later yields beauty, abundance, and growth.

Recall some "showers," or difficult seasons, you've gone through and reflect on the beauty that came out of those gloomy seasons. How did the tough times shape your perspective, grow your compassion, or help you better appreciate the goodness that came later on?

APRIL 20

Seek Out Some Blooms

Nature, Experience

Visit a local botanical garden or conservatory to admire the spring blooms! Snap a photo of just one special flower that catches your eye.

APRIL 21

Take What You Need

Self-Care

Take what you need, and carry it with you for the rest of your day:

- mindfulness of the energy you create and how it affects those around you
- mindfulness of what your body is telling you
- mindfulness of how the environment in which you spend your day affects you
- mindfulness of those around you who are facing challenges

APRIL 22

Set Your Soundtrack

Experience

Spend an entire day with instrumental music playing in the background. Whether it's classical compositions or scores from your favorite movies, let the music transport you and energize your day. Perhaps you'll find opportunities to replace the noise of the Top 40 hits on the radio, podcasts, or chatter from social media with instrumental classics.

APRIL 23

Nourish Yourself

Self-Care

Let food be thy medicine.

HIPPOCRATES (ATTRIBUTED)

A foundational component of living a full and vibrant life is eating foods that make you feel great.

Take a few minutes to reflect on what foods make you feel your best. This is not intended to be a list of the foods with healthy labels that proclaim to be good for you or the indulgent treats you enjoy in moderation. This is a closer look at what foods *actually* make your body feel energized and full of vitality when they're incorporated into your regular diet.

It's easy to fall into eating foods that are comforting, convenient, or even those based on the preferences of the people around you. Take some time today and throughout the next week to notice how you feel as you eat certain things and decide on a few foods that satiate your hunger, offer you vital nutrients, give you energy, and whose taste you enjoy. Plan out a few go-to meals that will help you feel your best.

APRIL 24
Prep a Springtime Quiche
Create

Take advantage of the springtime produce and prep a delicious breakfast to enjoy all week long!

Asparagus Quiche

Prep time: 15 minutes | Cook time: 45 minutes | Serves: 6

Ingredients

1 (9-inch) piecrust

$1/2$ tablespoon olive oil

$1/2$ cup sliced sweet onion

8 asparagus spears, ends removed and cut into 1-inch pieces

4 cups fresh baby spinach

5 large eggs

1 cup milk of choice

$3/4$ cup crumbled feta cheese

$1/4$ cup shredded mozzarella cheese

Salt and pepper, to taste

Instructions

1. Preheat the oven to 375 degrees Fahrenheit. Line a 9-inch pie plate with pie dough, and set it in the freezer while you prepare the filling.

2. In a large skillet, heat the olive oil over medium heat. Add the sliced onion, asparagus spears, and spinach. Cook until the asparagus spears are slightly tender and the spinach is wilted. Transfer the spinach to a colander. Press firmly with the back of a spoon to squeeze out as much liquid as possible. Set aside.

3. In a large bowl, whisk together the eggs and milk. Stir in the feta and mozzarella cheese. Season with salt and pepper, to taste.

4. Remove the piecrust from the freezer. Place the asparagus pieces, spinach, and onions on the bottom of the crust. Pour the egg and cheese mixture over the vegetables, filling the crust.

5. Bake for 45 minutes, or until the quiche is set and lightly golden brown. Let stand for 15 minutes before serving.

APRIL 25

Friendship

Whimsy, Connect

The flowers listed here communicated sentiments of friendship in the Victorian era.

zinnia: thoughts of absent friends, lasting affection

speedwell: feminine fidelity

ivy: affection, friendship, fidelity

arborvitae: unchanging friendship

jonquil: respect and friendship

periwinkle: blossoming friendship, "I hope we become friends"

Treat one of your friends to a specialty bouquet of flowers to thank them for all the ways they brighten your days.

APRIL 26

Give Sincere Thanks

Identity

In the end, maybe it's wiser to surrender before the miraculous
scope of human generosity and to just keep saying thank
you, forever and sincerely, for as long as we have voices.

ELIZABETH GILBERT, *Eat, Pray, Love*

APRIL 27

GIVE YOURSELF PERMISSION

Take Time to Prepare

Self-Care

Today give yourself permission to:

- spend time preparing for something in the future
- seek out advice from an expert on a topic you are unsure about
  (such as health, finances, career decisions, car maintenance)
- do the research you need in order to make an educated decision

APRIL 28

Give New Life to an Old Favorite

Home, Create

What item in your home could you reimagine to better fit the vibe you want to create? It's amazing what a fresh coat of paint or new hardware can do for an old piece of furniture. Check out the wide array of do-it-yourself videos online to find inspiration—and don't be afraid to experiment and have a little fun!

APRIL 29

Support a Charitable Cause

Identity, Experience

What charitable causes are you passionate about, interested in, or already familiar with? Jot down a list of volunteer work you've been exposed to in the past as well as avenues you may be interested in pursuing in the future.

Take a few minutes to research ways you can get involved, then determine what you are able to contribute right now based on their needs and your capacity. Your gift doesn't need to be tremendous or super time-consuming; every little bit helps.

APRIL 30

Strengthen Your Relationships and Community

Connect

> No man is an island, entire of itself;
> every man is a piece of the continent,
> a part of the main.

JOHN DONNE

The strength of any relationship is a direct result of how much effort is put into caring for it. To be emotionally connected with anyone—family, friends, or romantic partners—requires giving the gift of oneself. This doesn't mean grand gestures or exhaustive endeavors. Rather, it's about showing up with sincerity and consistency.

Take some time to think about the people in your life who show up for you in this way. What specifically do they do to make you feel seen and cared for? How might you return the favor in the days ahead?

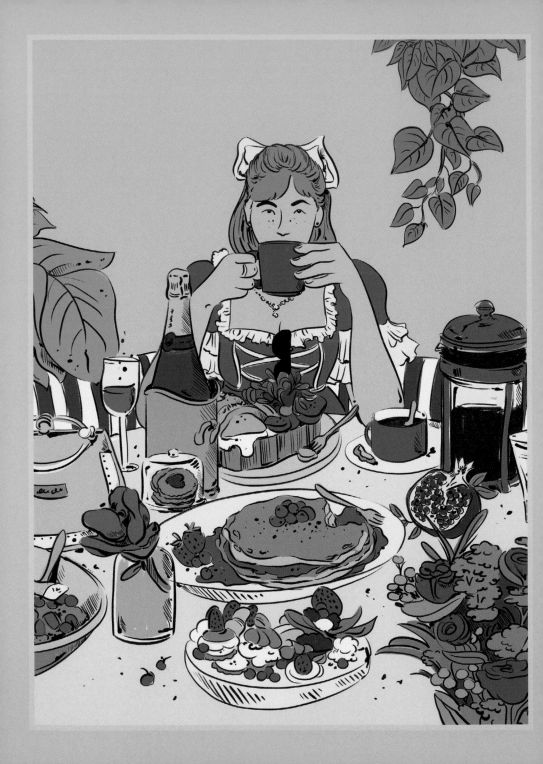

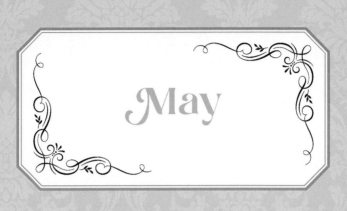

May

MAY 1

Wishing Tree

Connect, Whimsy, Create

Have you ever come across a wishing tree? It's one whose branches are decorated with dangling notes of prayers, hopes, and wishes that flutter in the wind. Start one in your city by writing a few of your own wishes on note cards and tying them with string to the branches of a tree. Leave a handful of empty cards, string, and markers to be used by passersby. While the notes won't last forever, this gesture will hopefully spark conversations that bring people together in your community.

MAY 2

Beauty Board

Create, Beauty

Dwell on the beauty of life.

MARCUS AURELIUS

Create a beauty vision board—a collage of things you find beautiful. Magazine clippings, photos, scraps of cards, quotes, and anything of beauty that inspires you in some way.

MAY 3

Breakfast Date

Experience

"When you wake up in the morning, Pooh," said Piglet at last,
"what's the first thing you say to yourself?"

"What's for breakfast?" said Pooh. "What do you say, Piglet?"

"I say, I wonder what's going to happen exciting today?" said
Piglet.

Pooh nodded thoughtfully. "It's the same thing," he said.

A. A. MILNE, *Winnie-the-Pooh*

Take yourself out for a leisurely breakfast—just because!

Whether it's a classic diner or a French café, this could be a fun way
to treat yourself and start your day off on a sweet note.

MAY 4
Reflect on Travel and
Coming Home to Yourself
Experience, Dream

Take a little thought journey with the wise words of Alain de Botton from *The Art of Travel*:

> Journeys are the midwives of thought. Few places are more conducive to internal conversations than moving planes, ships, or trains. There is an almost quaint correlation between what is before our eyes and the thoughts we are able to have in our heads: large thoughts at times requiring large views, and new thoughts, new places. Introspective reflections that might otherwise be liable to stall are helped along by the flow of the landscape. The mind may be reluctant to think properly when thinking is all it is supposed to do. . . .
>
> At the end of hours of train-dreaming, we may feel we have been returned to ourselves—that is, brought back into contact with emotions and ideas of importance to us. It is not necessarily at home that we best encounter our true selves.[11]

Outside of where you live, where are you most at home with yourself?

MAY 5
Recall Your Lightning-Strike Loves
Identity

———— FRENCH PHRASE OF THE DAY ————

Avoir un coup de foudre: falling in love at first sight; the literal translation is "to have a lightning strike"

It's likely that you've experienced a lightning-strike love in some shape or form. It may have been with a person who ended up being a great love or a great heartbreak. But it also may have been love at first sight with that pair of shoes you spotted and just knew they would make you feel so special when you slipped them on. Or perhaps with a pet when you first met. It may have been love at first taste with a new coffee blend over the winter. It may have been love at first listen with a song whose lyrics spoke just the right message you needed to hear. It may have been love at first conversation with that person with whom you would become best friends down the road.

What lightning-strike loves have you experienced? Grab your journal and see what you can recall. It's likely you'll have more than you would have expected!

MAY 6

Saving for Long-Term Goals

Self-Care, Dream

While long-term financial goals are less urgent than your immediate needs, they are no less important. Knowing what your long-term financial goals are will shape decisions you make in the short-term. While long-term goals often require budgeting and sacrifices, they will pay off!

What are some of your long-term financial goals? Jot them down, and don't be afraid to dream big!

MAY 7

Choose Your May Theme Song

Whimsy

The month of May conjures feelings of frolicking through fields of blossomed flowers in a billowing dress, hair tousled by the sun-warmed wind, eyes turned upward, and hopes dancing right at the heart's surface. Choose a theme song for this month that captures this feeling: wild and wide-open to the beauty of a world in bloom.

MAY 8

HELLO, LOVER

Hippophile

Whimsy

Hippophile: a lover of horses

In the world of animal spirits, the horse symbolizes nobility, trust, independence, movement, freedom, service, and alignment within one's mind, body, and spirit. Whether or not you're a bona fide hippophile, how can the majestic horse speak to you today?

MAY 9

Plan a Picnic

Connect, Experience

Plan a lovely picnic at the park with friends. Along with the snacks and drinks, don't forget to bring a deck of cards or portable game, a music speaker, bug spray to keep the pests away, and of course, sunscreen.

MAY 10
Million-Dollar Dreamer
Dream

What would you do if you won a million dollars?

Would you . . .

take an international vacation?

revamp your wardrobe?

buy a home?

indulge in a dream car, or maybe a dream boat?

start a philanthropic fund?

invest in that business idea you've been dreaming up?

Set aside ten minutes to indulge in the dreaming process.

While winning a million dollars may not be likely, let this practice guide some financial reach goals—those goals that can't be achieved without extra effort—as you continue to earn more. After brainstorming, take a look at your finances, and see how you can begin saving for your immediate needs as well as long-term dreams.

MAY 11
Bedding Refresh
Home, Self-Care, Coziness

To sleep, perchance to dream.

WILLIAM SHAKESPEARE, *Hamlet*

Who doesn't love jumping into clean, crisp bedding?

Consider this your reminder to wash your sheets, pillowcases, and outer comforter. But let's bring in a little romance: add a few drops of your favorite essential oil before tossing them in the dryer. Consider experimenting with lavender, ylang-ylang, sandalwood, or vanilla.

If your bed linens have seen better days, maybe it's time for a refresh! Declutter those nightstands, and put a little extra effort into making your bed a luxurious, cozy spot where you want to curl up at night and get your best sleep.

MAY 12
The Grass Is Always Greener
Whimsy

———————— ITALIAN PHRASE OF THE DAY ————————

L'erba del vicino è sempre più verde: the neighbor's grass is always greener.

The grass does always seem to be greener on the other side, does it not? The fact is that everyone—no matter their station or circumstance— deals with difficulties, and we must take care not to be disillusioned by the life of another, and not to compare.

To perhaps inspire you, there's another saying attributed to Neil Barringham:

"The grass is greener where you water it."

Better to tend that plot of land you call your own.

MAY 13

Photo Shoot

Identity, Create

Plan a styled photo shoot that encapsulates part of who you are. It could be at one of your favorite places, with your most treasured friends or a pet, doing a favorite hobby, or even enjoying a very *you* beverage. Wear clothes that make you feel like your truest self. Recruit a friend to take the photos, or set up a tripod and delight in the joy of this present moment in time—and create a tangible way to look back on it in the future.

MAY 14

Have Courage

Whimsy

Life shrinks or expands in proportion to one's courage.

ANAÏS NIN

How can you tap into a little more courage and expand your life today?

MAY 15

RECALIBRATE YOUR MORNING ROUTINE
Replenish Your Body's Water
Self-Care

Water is an essential nutrient, and your body can't produce enough of it on its own, so you need to hydrate throughout the day. While you sleep, your body continues using water without receiving a refill.

Starting your day with a glass of water not only replenishes your body's hydration after a night's rest, but it can also aid digestion, mental performance, and metabolism. Try adding a fresh squeeze of lemon juice for an added boost of polyphenols, antioxidants, and vitamin C.[12]

Or consider trying a fruit infusion by simply adding berries, cucumbers, melons, citrus, mint, or rosemary—or some combination thereof—to filtered water for some of the most deliciously refreshing recipes. You can find dozens of water infusion recipes online. Experiment to find your favorites, then garnish with fresh, ripe berries or mint to make it extra special.

MAY 16

Stand Out

Dream, Identity

No one ever made a difference by being like everyone else.

P. T. BARNUM, *The Greatest Showman*

What are some ways in which you wish you had the courage to be an even fuller version of yourself, even if that meant standing out from the crowd? Jot down your thoughts in a journal to reflect more deeply, and determine just one small way that you will choose to stand out—starting today!

MAY 17

Plant Summer Blooms

Home

Add some cheer to your home's outdoor space by planting summer blooms. Whether in flower boxes, pots, or flower beds, adding these pops of color is certain to brighten your mood and also add cheer to your corner of the neighborhood.

MAY 18

Dream a New Dream

Dream

You are never too old to set another goal or to dream a new dream.

LES BROWN, *Live Your Dreams*

MAY 19

Cultivate a New Habit

Self-Care, Experience

Today is a new day. Consider cultivating a new habit. Make the goal small and attainable, and just select one.

One way to help you cultivate your new habit is by creating a habit tracker. If you're more digitally inclined, use one of the many habit-tracking apps. Or if you're more analog, delve into the world of tracking with a bullet journal, or try a premade, already-designed habit tracker that you can purchase online. And if you're a hybrid, create your own inspiring tracker using a design app, then print and track your progress manually.

Embrace Small Beginnings

A journey of a thousand miles begins with a single step.

CHINESE PROVERB

Every journey begins with a first step. Whether you'd like to quit an undesirable habit or create new habits to support your goals, expert help abounds. To keep you focused on the path to creating a life you love, check out *Atomic Habits* by James Clear, *Tiny Habits* by B. J. Fogg, or *Mini Habits* by Stephen Guise.

Take What You Need

Take what you need, and carry it with you for the rest of your day:

- hopefulness
- patience
- creativity
- intentionality

HELLO, LOVER

Thalassophile

Whimsy

Thalassophile: a lover of the sea; someone who loves the sea, ocean

Not everyone lives near the ocean, but bringing elements of the ocean and sea life into your life can help remind you of their beauty and vastness.

And if you're a true thalassophile, how can you spread extra love to oceans this week? Perhaps getting involved in a beach cleanup? Or if you don't live near but still want to spread love, either make a donation to your favorite ocean cleanup initiatives or start right where you are and join a local blueway cleanup to help keep trash and debris out of your surrounding waterways.

MAY 23

Be a Lady of Leisure

Self-Care

Leisure has a value of its own. It is not a mere handmaid of labor; it is something we should know how to cultivate, to use, and to enjoy. It has a distinct and honorable place.

AGNES REPPLIER

Becoming a lady of leisure might be easier than you think.

Have you found yourself experiencing a midday slump? No worries. Simply peruse your home for a decorative pillow.

Next, settle into a comfortable chair, preferably next to a window.

Then place the pillow on a side table, ottoman, or whatever you can maneuver that will allow you to prop up your feet.

Now take a seat, bask in the afternoon light, and enjoy a few moments of fanciful pleasure. It's amazing what a little sunshine and feet propping will do.

MAY 24

Host a Spring Tasting Party

Connect

Coordinate a spring tasting party with your friends. It can be for any food or beverage you like. Either go for some of the regular choices, or think outside the box—all options are on the table! Here are some fun examples to try:

pastries and desserts

chicken salad

hummus

tea or coffee

wine or beer

cocktails or mocktails

cheese and crackers

After choosing the food item, have each guest bring a different variation or flavor of that item.

Line up the offerings and do a side-by-side tasting, comparing flavor notes, textures, and anything that makes sense for that food.

If you want to go the extra mile, look up tasting charts for the sampling item and provide copies at the party for everyone to reference. They may help you identify flavors that you hadn't noticed before.

MAY 25

Beauty

Whimsy

These are just a few flowers that communicated acknowledgments of beauty to the recipient in the Victorian era.

calla lily: beauty

hibiscus: delicate beauty

clematis: mental beauty

dwarf sunflower: adoration

Whether from a grocery store, flower shop, or your own backyard, select some flowers to arrange for yourself today. Place the arrangement on a table or countertop in your home, and allow yourself to delight in its beauty throughout the coming days. When you notice the petals beginning to droop, select one flower from the arrangement. Press it between absorbent sheets of paper, and place it between the pages of your favorite book. When you revisit this title in years to come and happen upon the preserved beauty of this little flower, give thanks for your ability to appreciate such a simple yet timeless treasure.

MAY 26

Read Romantic Movement Poetry

Whimsy, Experience

Gain another view into the origins of the Romantic movement. Look up works from the well-known English Romantic poets, such as William Wordsworth, Samuel Taylor Coleridge, John Keats, Percy Bysshe Shelley, William Blake, and Lord Byron.

MAY 27

Anticipate Summer Travels

Whimsy

——— SWEDISH WORD OF THE DAY ———

Resfeber: the restlessness in a traveler's heart before a journey begins; a "travel fever" of anxiety and anticipation

Do you have any upcoming travel to get excited about? If travel isn't currently on your horizon, how can you tap into some *resfeber* by planning a local trip or outing near you?

MAY 28
Savor Noteworthy Words
Create

Start a running list of your favorite quotes. Quotes from people you admire, quotes that inspire you, quotes that make you think differently. Keep these in a journal, on a Pinterest board, or in a notes document on your phone or computer—somewhere you can continue to add to and reference later.

MAY 29
Visit a Beekeeper
Experience

The process of bees making honey is a fascinating one, as is the relationship between bees and their beekeepers.

Get a firsthand lesson in how honey is made by visiting a local farm or beekeeper, and pick up a jar of the sweet stuff while you're there. As an added benefit, honey is believed to help with specific conditions, including cough, wound care, cardiovascular disease, gastrointestinal disease, and neurological disease.[13]

MAY 30
Try an Outdoor Exercise Class
Experience, Nature

As temperatures warm up, a variety of free or low-cost exercise classes are offered outside. From yoga to circuit training, engaging in outdoor exercise is a great way to be active while also mixing up your normal routine—not to mention, getting some vitamin D.

If you need some help getting started, here are some ideas for exercise classes and group activities to get you moving more outdoors:

yoga in the park or at a beach

circuit training

trail running groups

kayaking or rowing groups

walking and hiking meetups

group cycling

tennis

swimming and water aerobics

skiing, snowboarding, and snowshoeing

Which ones call to you? Look up what outdoor exercise classes or group meetups are being offered in your community, and try out a new one.

MAY REFLECTIONS

Invigorate Your Creative Energy

Create

Creativity takes courage.

HENRI MATISSE

In a consumer-driven culture, it can be easy to succumb to distractions. But if we don't guard our time, energy, and attention, we can allow our unique gifts of creativity to be wasted.

Looking back at the last month, how much time did you spend watching rather than doing?

How much did you consume rather than create?

You are uniquely and wonderfully made, and your creativity is an expression of the depth of this magic. Think about how you can create—and celebrate—more in the days ahead.

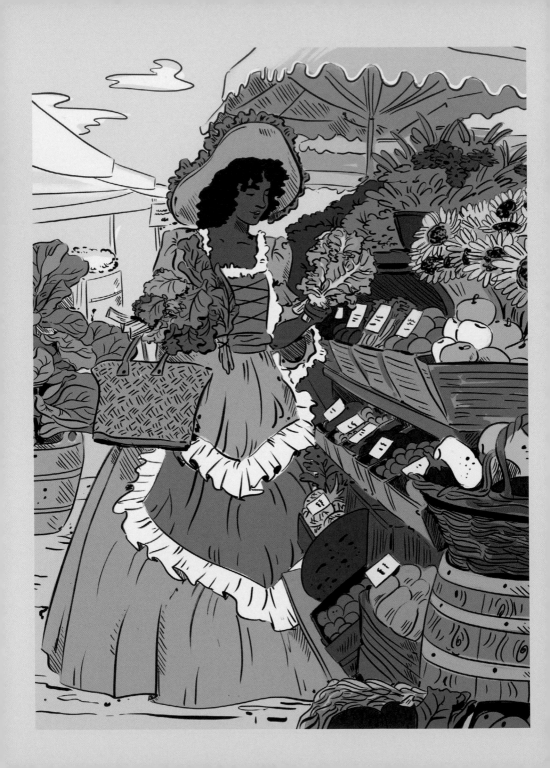

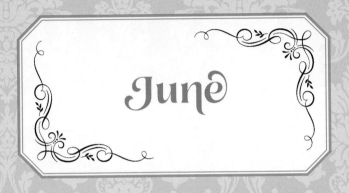

June

JUNE 1

Farmers Market

Experience

Forgo your usual trip to the grocery store and head to a farmers market instead! Grab your produce for the week, a fresh bouquet of flowers, and strike up a conversation with some of the vendors to learn about the personal stories behind their businesses.

JUNE 2

Find Your Summer Scent

Beauty, Identity

Find your signature summer scent. Do some exploring and find something that complements this season of nostalgia, relaxation, and light-heartedness. Look for scents with notes of freshly cut grass, citrus fruit trees, bergamot, citronella, or full florals like jasmine, rose, and geranium. Whether in a perfume, body lotion, or a scent for your home, find something that smells like a summer breeze at sunset.

JUNE 3

Honor Your Calling Without Fear

Dream

How very little can be done under the spirit of fear.

FLORENCE NIGHTINGALE

Despite being born into a wealthy upbringing in 1820, Florence Nightingale felt pulled to enter the field of nursing—an occupation that was reserved for the lower classes, and definitely not for women.

Driven by faith and compelled to care for those in need, Florence began her career as a nurse at age thirty, studying in hospitals throughout Europe. She became superintendent of the Institution for the Care of Sick Gentlewomen in distressed circumstances in London, where her handling of the cholera epidemic caught the attention of the British government, who asked her to serve at a military hospital in Turkey where the army was fighting the Crimean War. Not far from the front line, Florence cared for injured soldiers, saving countless lives.[14]

Florence's compassion, wisdom, and courage made her a national heroine. Not only did she go on to institute major hygienic improvements and general practices in medical care, but Florence was integral in changing the perception of nursing into an admirable and sought-after professional calling.

Is fear holding you back from a cause or calling that you feel inspired to pursue? How might Florence's bravery and compassion inspire you to pursue a worthy purpose in your own life?

JUNE 4
Host a "Lemonade" Stand
Whimsy, Connect

Host your own free pop-up stand! Pick a high-traffic spot, make a fun sign, set up your table, and serve whatever strikes your fancy. Maybe it's the traditional lemonade, or perhaps it's infused water, cookies, pastries, or popsicles.

Hand out these goodies for free and enjoy bringing unexpected delight to people's day!

JUNE 5
Summertime Affirmations
Self-Care, Identity

How did your springtime affirmations go? Did you commit to looking at the list daily? Whether you stuck with it or need a fresh start, spend some time thinking about your affirmations for this summer season. As the weather warms and days stretch out, what affirming or hopeful words do you need to speak to yourself every day?

JUNE 6

Plan a Pool Day

Experience, Whimsy

As temperatures begin to warm up, what better way to kick off the summer spirit than a pool day? Grab some fun snacks, sun protection, your favorite float, and a colorful beach towel and you'll be ready to roll. Invite some friends (or grab a book or some magazines) and enjoy a few hours soaking up the sun!

And if it's still a little chilly where you live, maybe use this time to start planning some epic pool adventures. Don't have a pool of your own? No worries; find a local community pool or use an app to find a pool or hot tub to rent for the afternoon.

JUNE 7

Choose Your June Theme Song

Whimsy

Summertime is here and that means windows down, shoes off, and living easy. Choose a June theme song that sounds like salt in the air and cares tossed to the wind.

JUNE 8
Enjoy a Simple Summer Salad
Create

This simple salad makes a perfect side dish for a potluck picnic or a weeknight dinner at home—and it comes together in a snap!

Summer Salad
Prep time: 10 minutes | Serves: 4

Ingredients

1 English cucumber, sliced

2 to 3 ripe tomatoes, diced

$1/2$ red onion, chopped

2 tablespoons olive oil

1 tablespoon red wine vinegar

Salt and pepper, to taste

1 tablespoon fresh herbs (optional)

Instructions

1. Toss all the ingredients in a bowl.
2. Chill for 20 minutes, then enjoy.

JUNE 9

Buy Some Sunnies

Whimsy

Buy some new sunglasses to wear all summer long! Fun, colorful, chic, retro—whatever strikes your fancy.

JUNE 10

Show Some Love

Connect

———— ITALIAN SAYING OF THE DAY ————

L'amore e la fede dall'opera si vede.
Translation: Love and faith can be seen from the work.

As we all know, loving friends and family isn't always easy, especially during stressful circumstances like heartache, enduring health challenges, or going through major life changes.

Think about someone in your life who is taking a bit of extra energy to love well right now. Reflect on how you met, all of the qualities you love about them, and the fun memories you've shared. Then dream up some of the ways you can show up for them, offer them support, or make their burden a little lighter during this season.

JUNE 11

Plan a Day Trip

Experience

As summer settles in, often so does the craving for a little getaway. Plan a day trip somewhere within a few hours of your home and enjoy a change in atmosphere.

JUNE 12

Grow an Herb Garden

Experience

Herbs are not only packed with flavor, but they are also loaded with nutrients and antioxidants that have amazing benefits for your health. Rather than buying pricey packages of herbs that spoil quickly, pick up a few small plants to have on hand all summer long. Keep them on your kitchen counter or plant them in pots outside. Adding these fresh herbs to pastas, salads, marinades, and many other dishes can really take them to the next level.

JUNE 13

Raise Your Voice

Identity

When the whole world is silent, even one voice becomes powerful.

MALALA YOUSAFZAI, Pakistani female education
activist and 2014 Nobel Peace Prize laureate

JUNE 14

Dive into Your Fascination of the Month

Self-Care

What's the thing that you're currently fascinated by? That topic you can't learn enough about. Gardening, fashion, music composition, international politics, or sustainable living?

Set some goals to help you dive more deeply into whatever it is. Aim to read three books on the topic, watch interviews with ten experts, or start a blog to document what you're learning.

JUNE 15

RECALIBRATE YOUR MORNING ROUTINE

Start Your Day with a Healthy Meal

Self-Care

Starting your day with a healthy, protein-rich breakfast can help increase your energy and reduce your cravings throughout the hours ahead. Instead of grabbing a granola bar as you race out the door, leave some extra time in the morning to nourish your body with a delicious meal. Maybe even keep a special dish or bowl reserved specifically for breakfast so that you can enjoy an added touch of elegance with your first meal of the day.

JUNE 16

Create Beauty in Humility

Whimsy, Beauty

The humblest tasks get beautified if loving hands do them.

LOUISA MAY ALCOTT, *Little Women*

JUNE 17
Print Your Memories
Create

There's something special about seeing your memories in print. You could print them out and put them in an old-fashioned album, scrapbook them, or design a photo book online and have it printed.

Don't succumb to the pressure to only print the "mountaintop moment" pictures. Print your everyday memories that brought a smile to your face: that classic car you snapped a picture of, the rainbow that colored the sky after the huge storm, that screenshot you took of a text conversation that made you laugh out loud. Archive and celebrate these magical everyday moments that brought you joy.

JUNE 18
Just Buy the Flowers
Beauty, Nature, Self-Care

This is your excuse to just buy the flowers this week. Grab that bouquet from the grocery store, or pop into a local flower shop. Treat yourself to this small gift that will brighten up your space in a big way.

JUNE 19

Beauty Maker

Beauty, Identity

I want to make everything around me beautiful, and
that will be my life.

ELSIE DE WOLFE

Elsie de Wolfe, also known as Lady Mendl, was the first professional deco-
rator in the United States. An innovator and style icon, the risks she took
forever changed the direction of interior decor and continue to live on
today.[15]

While this well-known statement of hers is often thought of in terms
of interior design, this outlook can apply to a way of existing in the
world, wanting to make *everything* around you beautiful. Stretching far
beyond decor, this desire to cultivate beauty applies to relationships,
workplaces, neighborhoods, and ultimately the impact you leave on the
world.

How will you beautify the things within your sphere of influence?

JUNE 20

Hydrate

Self-Care

Giving your body the water it needs is essential to feeling your best. Doctors often recommend drinking the number of ounces that is equivalent to your weight in pounds, divided by two. For example: 140 pounds, divided by 2, results in 70 ounces of water a day.[16] But, of course, check with your doctor about what amount of water intake is best for you.

If you struggle to stay hydrated, try some new tactics. Treat yourself to a new water bottle—one that you like to look at and hold—and carry it with you throughout the day, set a timer on your phone to remind you to drink, or try hydrating with water infused with refreshing lemon or cucumber.

JUNE 21

Promenade

Create, Connect, Self-Care

Dress up in an extra chic outfit—just because! Take a stroll in your Sunday best. Or simply go out for a drink with a friend or take yourself on a solo date.

JUNE 22
Take What You Need
Whimsy, Self-Care

Take what you need to carry into today:

- permission to take a break to do something to care for your needs—physical, emotional, or mental
- permission to turn to an old favorite rather than try something new
- permission to admit you were wrong
- permission to reevaluate something that isn't serving you

JUNE 23
Ponder *Sonder*
Whimsy

———— ENGLISH WORD OF THE DAY ————

Sonder: The profound feeling of realizing that everyone, including strangers passing in the street, has a life as complex as one's own, which they are constantly living despite one's personal lack of awareness of it.

JUNE 24

Summer Stargazing

Nature, Experience

Grab some friends and go stargazing. Look up what constellations you should be able to see based on your location and time of year, as well as the astrological stories that go along with them.

JUNE 25

FLORIOGRAPHY LESSON

Encouragement

Whimsy

Who could use encouragement today? Consider bringing someone a bouquet of flowers to help them feel supported and cared for. Below is a list of a few flowers that communicated sentiments of encouragement during the Victorian era:

chamomile: patience in adversity

goldenrod: encouragement, good fortune

dark crimson rose: mourning

JUNE 26

Ailurophile

Whimsy

Ailurophile: a lover of cats

Not everyone is a bona fide ailurophile. Perhaps you've heard of *Old Possum's Book of Practical Cats* by T. S. Eliot, on which Andrew Lloyd Webber's *Cats* was based. A lesser-known book, *The Book of Cats* by Charles H. Ross, also delves into the realm of all-things cats for those who can't get enough of our feline friends:

> The Chinese look into their Cat's eyes to know what o'clock it is; and the playfulness of Cats is said to indicate the coming of a storm. I have noticed this often myself and have seen them rush about in a half wild state just before windy weather. I think it is when the wind is *rising* that they are most affected.

ROMANTICISM LESSON

Admire Romantic Movement Art

Whimsy, Experience

Head to your local art museum, or peruse museums online, and admire art from the Romantic movement. Expressions of the movement will vary based on the region the artist was creating. See if you can pick up on these nuances:

- German Romantic painters focused on interior emotions instead of reasoned observations. They looked to previous eras, including the Middle Ages, for examples of men living in harmony with nature and each other.
- Spanish Romantic painters began exploring more subjective views of landscapes and portraits, valorizing the individual.
- French artists had a larger repertoire of subjects that included portraiture and history painting, and also developed a sculptural rendition of Romanticism.
- English Romantic painters, not as dramatic as their German counterparts, favored landscape. Their depictions were more naturalistic and often practiced en plein air painting.
- American Romanticism found its primary expression in landscape painting, emphasizing awe at the vastness of nature.

JUNE 28

Share Mango Salsa

Create

This salsa is perfect for a cookout—and great served with tortilla chips or on top of grilled chicken, steak, or fish.

Mango Salsa

Prep time: 30 minutes | Serves: 6

Ingredients

3 large ripe mangoes (or 6 small ripe mangoes), peeled and diced

2 ripe avocados, diced

1 red bell pepper, chopped

1 jalapeño pepper, diced, with seeds removed

1 (15-ounce) can black beans, drained and rinsed

2 tablespoons fresh lime juice

1 to 2 tablespoons honey, to taste

Salt, to taste

Instructions

1. Toss in a bowl the mangoes, avocados, and peppers, then mix in the black beans.
2. Add in the lime juice and a drizzle of honey. You can play with the amounts of these ingredients—add to your liking.
3. Finally, add a sprinkle of salt, and enjoy!

JUNE 29
Find Your City's Best
Experience

Set out on a quest this summer to find your city's "best of" something! It could be the best local bookstore, sushi restaurant, roadside farm stand, or rock climbing gym. Use this as an opportunity to explore and sample local gems you might have previously overlooked.

JUNE 30
JUNE REFLECTIONS
Nurture an Environment for Yourself and Others
Home

Your home is an expression of your unique makeup: your values, your personality, your needs, and your contributions to others. As you look around your home today, does it feel like an accurate expression of you? Reflecting on the past month, have you stewarded this gift of your home well? How can you make it feel more nurturing for yourself and for the people who walk through your door?

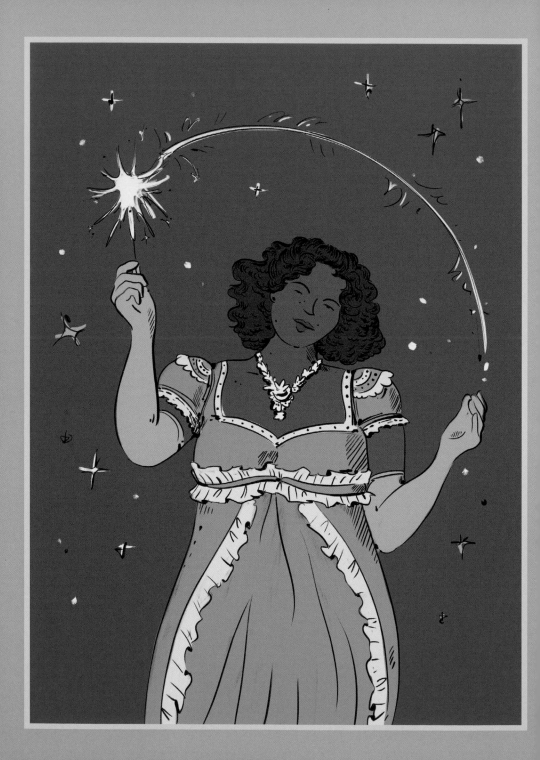

July

JULY 1

True to Yourself

Identity, Dream

From now on, I'm going to own myself and be true to myself. I no longer want to live someone else's idea of what and who I should be. I am going to be me.

DIANA, Princess of Wales

JULY 2

Infused Water

Self-Care, Experience

The heat of summer calls for spa-worthy infused water. Chop up a handful of your favorite fruits and herbs, toss them in a pitcher of water, and chill it in the fridge to enjoy all day.

Strawberries and basil, cucumbers and watermelon, blueberries and thyme—there are endless refreshing flavor combinations to make your daily hydration just a little more fun.

JULY 3
Make a List of Your Wild Things
Dream

Make a list of the wildest, most adventurous things you've done. Then make a list of the wild and adventurous things you'd like to try. Which one can you knock off that bucket list next?

JULY 4
Sparkly Nights
Experience, Connect

Buy a few sparklers and invite some friends over to delight in those magical sparks of light! Dance, laugh, enjoy, and celebrate this gift of freedom.

JULY 5
Confront Your Inner Critic
Self-Care

Every person has inner voices of self-doubt, criticisms, and what-ifs. Even those now labeled as successful had to navigate their own inner critics throughout their journeys.

Turn the tables on yourself, and do some evaluating. What are your inner critic's go-to critical remarks, stinging words, and downright mean comments? Identifying these falsities and self-doubts will help you spot them as they pop up throughout your day. Pinpointing your inner critic's most reliable lies will help prevent you from getting this negativity confused with your own inner voice of hope, determination, and courage to pursue the life you feel called to.

JULY 6
Enjoy a Summertime Sweet
Experience, Connect

Take a friend out for a summertime treat. Whether it's a toppling ice cream cone, fruity slushy, or slice of peach cobbler from the farmers market, enjoy an evening outside with some uniquely summer flavors.

JULY 7
Choose Your July Theme Song
Whimsy

In summer, the song sings itself.

WILLIAM CARLOS WILLIAMS, "The Botticellian Trees"

For this month's theme song, why not try composing the lyrics yourself? Write a poem that captures how summer feels to you—from the hazy days of adolescent memories to what you see, hear, taste, and feel in this very moment of the present. Find a dreamy instrumental track to provide the perfect background to your poetry.

JULY 8
Sunset Drive
Experience, Self-Care

Head out on a sunset drive—one with expansive views that will allow you to see far across the horizon for an unimpeded look at the evening sky. Turn on a playlist that strikes the right mood, and soak up that gorgeous golden-hour light.

JULY 9

Toss a Coin in a Fountain

Whimsy, Experience

The tradition of fountain coin tosses can be traced back to ancient civilizations. Without modern plumbing and water filtration methods, sources of drinking water were viewed as gifts from the gods. As cities' infrastructure became more advanced and fountains were built, a small statue of an ancient god was often placed next to the fountains, turning them into a shrine of sorts, where people would say prayers as they collected their drinking water.[17]

While fountains are no longer our source of clean drinking water, the joy of the coin toss and a little wish lives on. Find a scenic fountain in your city, toss in a coin, and make a wish.

JULY 10

Act Out of Hope

Dream, Connect

May your choices reflect your hopes, not your fears.

NELSON MANDELA (ATTRIBUTED),
first president of South Africa

JULY 11

Watch Fireflies

Nature, Beauty, Whimsy

Head outside as dusk begins to settle in, and search for fireflies to watch as they flash and flit. Listen to the sounds of evening settling down, and relax into the gentle gift of one day that has passed and another that will begin anew in the morning.

JULY 12

BECOME A FINANCE QUEEN

Nice-to-Haves

Self-Care

When you're working to save for a long-term goal or have a financial need pop up, items in the nice-to-have category are what can be scaled back first. These often include dining out, entertainment, clothing, and travel for leisure.

Are there any nice-to-haves that you can scale back to devote more savings elsewhere? As an added bonus, when you develop a mindset that allows luxuries to be a treat rather than the norm, you'll appreciate those sweet rewards that much more.

JULY 13
Mini Backyard Makeover
Home, Create

Do a mini makeover of the outdoor spaces around your home. Whether it's a backyard, front porch, apartment balcony, or shared communal garden, how might you be able to better use this space? Would it help to place a selection of candles to add ambience at night? Bug spray to have on hand to keep pests away? If you're using a shared space, use this as an opportunity to connect with your neighbors and make this a fun community-building project.

JULY 14
Enjoy an Outdoor Concert
Experience

Enjoy an outdoor concert. Summertime offers an abundance of free options, ranging from local singers to orchestras to a cappella choirs.

JULY 15

RECALIBRATE YOUR MORNING ROUTINE

Fancify Your Morning Beverage

Self-Care

Who says you have to pay a fortune for a fancy coffee? You can make a delicious specialty coffee or tea in your very own kitchen. An affordable handheld frother can transform milk into delectable foam that will make your morning brew feel like a delightful treat that beckons you to get out of bed and greet the day.

JULY 16

HELLO, LOVER

Retrophile

Whimsy

Retrophile: a person who loves artifacts and aesthetics from the past

Consider visiting an antique store or vintage shop and see what speaks to you from another time and place.

JULY 17
Draw with Sidewalk Chalk
Whimsy, Create

Grab a box of sidewalk chalk and doodle away. Draw a nature scene or beautiful patterns, or write some encouraging phrases for those who pass by.

JULY 18
Drink Out of a Fancy Glass
Whimsy

A fancy glass makes a drink more fun. If you don't have one that feels set apart from what's currently in your cupboard, browse through a local shop and find one that strikes your fancy. It could be an antique teacup, champagne flute, or even a tiki mug—just pick something that feels special to you.

JULY 19

Feel the Earth Beneath Your Feet

Nature

Head to a grassy area and kick off your shoes. Feel the cool grass under your bare feet, and delight in this physical connection with the earth.

JULY 20

Don't Take It for Granted

Beauty, Self-Care

Until I feared I would lose it, I never loved to read.
One does not love breathing.

HARPER LEE, *To Kill a Mockingbird*

Spend some time reflecting on the gifts in your life that you love but may be taking for granted. Which activities, comforts, and—most importantly— people could you do a better job of cherishing and appreciating?

JULY 21
Take What You Need
Whimsy, Self-Care

Depending on where you live, this could be that time during summer where days grow long and the combination of sunshine plus heat and humidity can really begin to zap your energy. Perhaps you need a little pick-me-up today.

Take what you need, and carry it with you for the rest of your day:

- sparkle
- lightness
- excitement
- pizzazz
- vitality
- moxie
- dazzle

JULY 22
Reflections on Staying and Going
Self-Care, Identity

Deciding whether to stick with a chosen path or change direction can be a tough decision-making process. Carve out a few minutes to journal about decisions you've had to make in the past, gathering lessons learned in one place to inform the way you make decisions in the future.

Reflect on the following questions:

- What are some instances when you chose to stick with something despite challenges, losing enthusiasm, or a shift in priorities? Are you glad you stayed, or do you wish you had walked away sooner?
- What are some instances when you chose to walk away from something due to challenges, losing enthusiasm, or a change in priorities? Are you glad you walked away when you did, or do you wish you had stuck with it longer?
- Is there anything you are considering sticking with or walking away from right now? Perhaps this reflection might have some impact on your future decision-making.

JULY 23

Go on a Sunset Walk

Nature

Take advantage of the longer, warmer days, and go on an after-dinner sunset walk. Admire the warmth of the golden, pink, and lavender sky tones as they shift. Listen to the humming of the cicadas and chirping of crickets. Look out for fireflies as they sparkle across the grass and for other wildlife that may be emerging for the evening.

JULY 24

Sail Away

Experience, Nature

You don't have to set sail into the great unknown, but why not ride the waves for a few hours? Most cities with bodies of water nearby have places to rent sailboats, rowboats, canoes, kayaks, or paddleboards. Check out what's available in your area, and take to the water for a day!

JULY 25

Affirmations

Whimsy

Below is a list of flowers that affirm special and specific virtues the sender sees in the recipient.

Who in your life could use a little encouragement? Who in your life inspires you? Perhaps you could offer them just the message they need in the form of one of these blooms.

lily of the valley: happiness, sweetness
crocus: cheerfulness
edelweiss: courage
angelica: inspiration
iris: faith, trust, wisdom, hope, valor
calla lily: magnificent beauty
amethyst: admiration
yellow jasmine: elegance and grace
garden sage: esteem

JULY 26

GIVE YOURSELF PERMISSION

Get Those Documents in Order

Self-Care

Today give yourself permission to organize those important documents that you never need until you *really* need them. These might be for your home, vehicle, retirement, employment, or taxes. Store them in filing folders, and either scan or take photos of them for digital storage as well. It may feel like a tedious task, but it's an important one, and your future self will thank you!

JULY 27

Make a Creativity List

Home, Create

Make a list of things you would like to create. This could range from home projects to more artistic ideas you have brewing. Keep the running list in a memorable spot so you can refer back to it when you feel inspired to work on a project.

JULY 28

Paint En Plein Air

Create, Experience

All pictures painted inside in the studio will never be as
good as the things done outside.

PAUL CÉZANNE

Tap into your creative side while also enjoying the outdoors by painting
(or drawing) en plein air.

En plein air is a French expression meaning "in the open air," and
refers to the act of painting outdoors with the subject in full view. Plein
air artists strive to capture the spirit and essence of a landscape or
subject by incorporating natural light, color, and movement into their
works.

For examples, look to some of the more notable artists and advocates
in this discipline, such as Claude Monet, Camille Pissarro, Alfred Sisley,
Pierre-Auguste Renoir, Mary Cassatt, Vincent van Gogh, and Edgar Payne.
You'll notice a variety of styles, subjects, and colors used, meaning there's
no one right way.

Regardless of how advanced your artistic skills are, give it a try!

JULY 29

Always Be Whimsical

Whimsy, Identity

You must never ever stop being whimsical. And you must
not, ever, give anyone else the responsibility for your life.

MARY OLIVER, *Wild Geese*

JULY 30

Make Friendship Bracelets

Create, Connect

Tap into some summer nostalgia by making friendship bracelets. Pick
up yarn, beads, and charms, then invite a few friends over, and braid
away. Swap bracelets to wear for the rest of the summer, just like the
good old days.

JULY 31

JULY REFLECTIONS

Seek Out Newness and Adventure

Experience

> I could tell you my adventures beginning from this
> morning . . . but it's no use going back to yesterday,
> because I was a different person then.

LEWIS CARROLL, *Alice's Adventures in Wonderland*

While there is great joy found in the habitual delights of every day, there is also nothing like breaking from your routine to challenge yourself and grow. Newness doesn't have to be scary, and adventure doesn't have to require a big budget. Sometimes it means just stepping out your front door, perhaps walking in a new direction.

Looking back over the last month, did you do anything to get outside your comfort zone? If so, what did you learn about yourself or about the world? If not, how can you seek out some kind of adventure in the days ahead?

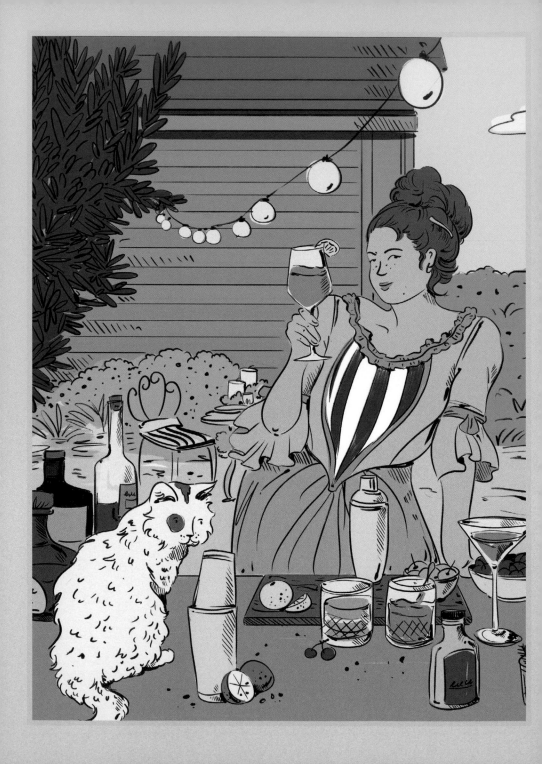

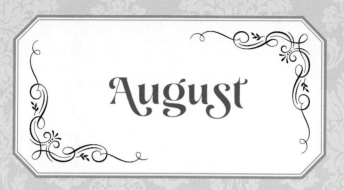

August

AUGUST 1
Your Happy Place
Whimsy, Self-Care

───────────── SPANISH WORD OF THE DAY ─────────────

Querencia: a place from which one's strength is drawn, where one feels secure and at home; the place where you are your most authentic self

From where do you draw your strength? Is it with a particular person or with a group of people? Is it through spending time alone? Is it when you're creating, or learning, or using the skills and experiences you have to help others? Take a moment to tap into your own *querencia* and get a healthy dose of strength for today.

AUGUST 2
Host a Movie Night
Connect, Home

Host an at-home movie night with a group of friends! Keep it simple or go all out with snacks that match the movie's theme. Maybe even show a double-feature. Or consider a weekly film series for those film franchises that have three or more movies.

AUGUST 3
Put Yourself in the Path of Beauty
Beauty

My mother would always say, no matter how hard things are, no matter how miserable or ugly things seem in your life on any given day, you always have the opportunity to put yourself in the way of beauty. There's always a sunrise and there's always a sunset, and it's up to you to be there for it or not.

CHERYL STRAYED, author of *Wild: From Lost to Found on the Pacific Crest Trail*

What are some ways that you can put yourself in the path of beauty, even on your hardest days? Beautiful places, beautiful things, beautiful words, beautiful souls.

Become a beauty seeker in your own life. Jot down a list of all things beautiful in your journal to refer back to on hard days or during hard seasons.

AUGUST 4
Sketch Your Dream House
Create, Dream

Everyone has some version of a dream home. Whether it's an apartment in a certain city, a home of their very own, or a large estate decked out with amenities like a pool, greenhouse, or tennis court.

Take a pen to paper, and write out the qualities you'd want in your dream home. If drawing is something you enjoy, begin sketching out your ideas. If collaging inspiration pics is more your style, start a dream board for your dream home.

AUGUST 5
Find a Sunflower Patch
Whimsy

Sunflowers are at their peak in late summer, with some varieties growing over ten feet tall! Look up where the closest sunflower patches are to you. Drive by, maybe stop and snap some pics with friends, or just enjoy a morning walk through the fields of joyful blooms.

AUGUST 6

Style Yourself

Identity, Create

Style is a way to say who you are without having to speak.

RACHEL ZOE (ATTRIBUTED), fashion
designer, businesswoman, and author

Instead of simply getting dressed today, think about what you want to communicate through your attire. Then dress accordingly!

AUGUST 7

Choose Your August Theme Song

Whimsy

Summer will soon fade into fall. With its end, a new beginning. Choose a theme song that mourns the melancholic beauty of an impending good-bye or celebrates the anticipation of a fresh start.

AUGUST 8

Accept the Fluidity of Joy

Whimsy, Self-Care

We dream of a durable kind of happiness, a state of bliss that, once found, has the constancy of granite. And while there are many things we can do to create a reservoir of joy that helps us amplify the highs and buffer the lows of everyday life, sometimes we have to accept that joy moves through our lives in an unpredictable way.

INGRID FETELL LEE, *Joyful: The Surprising Power of Ordinary Things to Create Extraordinary Happiness*

AUGUST 9

Create a Reservoir of Joy List

Whimsy, Self-Care

What are the activities that add to your reservoir of joy? What recharges your batteries, leaves you feeling refreshed, inspires you, or brightens your outlook? Make a list of these activities that you can refer back to when you're feeling down or depleted.

AUGUST 10
A Reason for Being
Dream, Identity

———— JAPANESE WORD OF THE DAY ————

Ikigai: a reason for being; an encompassing purpose, passion, and joy that gives an individual satisfaction and a sense of meaning in life

According to ikigai-living.com, when translated, *iki* means "life" and *kai* (or *gai)* means "reason."[18] The site offers several other loose translations in English, and here are a few that might resonate with you as you're romanticizing your life:

- the meaning of life
- happiness of being
- what makes life worth living

The Japanese concept of *ikigai* provides a holistic way to view one's life that includes one's passions, what the world needs, what one is good at, and what one can be paid for.[19]

Look up an ikigai chart online and start filling one out for yourself. You'll quickly see that the key to a fulfilling life isn't having everything fall into all four categories. Rather, a diverse array of pursuits lays a foundation for a full and balanced life.

AUGUST 11

Evaluate the Treasure You've Been Desiring

Identity

It's amazing how easy it can be to idealize another person's life—their talent, their career, their family, their belongings. But everything in life comes with a cost. When looking at someone else's life from the outside, we often lose sight of that reality.

Where have you sensed jealousy sneaking into your thoughts recently? Now reflect on the time, resources, and sacrifices required for someone to have "that thing" that has sparked your envy. If you could, would you choose to make the sacrifices required to have what they have? Or does this give you a sense of gratitude for your own life?

AUGUST 12

GIVE YOURSELF PERMISSION

Organize Your Personal Space

Self-Care

Today give yourself permission to organize a part of your home that only you see but that will make your days easier.

AUGUST 13

Be Your Own Bartender

Create, Beauty

Teach yourself how to make a fancy summer drink, one that's appealing to the eyes and the taste buds. Summer spritzes, juices, alcohol-free fizzes, margaritas—your options are endless!

Whatever you do, don't skip the garnish and special glass; presentation goes a long way!

AUGUST 14

You Be the Artist

Dream

Imagine: If you were commissioned to create a piece of art that aligned with the Romantic movement, what would you create?

A painting?

A sculpture?

A poem?

What would the subject be? With which Romantic artist would you want to apprentice?

AUGUST 15

Stretch It Out

Self-Care

Just like your body needs rest and recovery, movement is needed to reduce stiffness and boost circulation as your body wakes up for the day ahead. Look up a few simple morning stretches online, and try integrating these into your morning routine.

AUGUST 16

Be Fairy Godmother for a Day

Whimsy, Dream, Connect

If you could be a friend's fairy godmother for a day, what would you do for this person? Dream up some big ideas (and little ideas) for how each of your closest friends might feel the most cared for, and jot them down in a journal. Keep this stock of fairy dust on hand for this friend's next birthday or whenever he or she needs a pick-me-up!

AUGUST 17

Swing the Night Away

Experience

After dinner, once the day's heat dies down, head to a local playground and just swing.

AUGUST 18

Write a Note to Your Younger Self

Self-Care

Writing a note to your younger self can be a therapeutic experience and help you cultivate self-compassion. Think of yourself at a specific age. What would you tell that person? What have you learned since you were her age? In what ways are you proud of her? Journal a note to your younger self, extending compassion and offering wisdom and encouragement based on what you have learned over time.

AUGUST 19
Plan a Game Night
Connect

Plan a game night with friends, neighbors, or acquaintances you would like to get to know better. Invite guests to bring their favorite game to give your group a variety to choose from. It's amazing how a bit of fun competition brings out different sides of people's personalities.

AUGUST 20
Organize Your Drawers
Home

Whether it's a dresser drawer, kitchenware drawer, or that one random drawer where everything without an assigned place gets tossed, select a drawer you use daily that could be better organized. Take the time to make it neat and orderly, and you'll be glad you did when you revisit it in the days to come.

AUGUST 21
Take What You Need
Whimsy, Self-Care

We all need a little courage from time to time, and courage can take many different forms. Think about who are some of the most courageous people you know, whether they're famous or from your own life. Even if you are already steadfast in your courage, perhaps there's some area where an extra dose of courage can make a difference.

Take what you need, and carry it with you for the rest of your day:

- courage to embrace a new dream
- courage to try a new style, even if you don't think it will stick forever
- courage to show yourself grace in an area of life that is frustrating
- courage to believe in new beginnings and unexpected opportunities
- courage to try for that dream job
- courage to meet someone new
- courage to say the difficult things
- courage to listen to something you'd rather not hear

AUGUST 22
Organize a Weekly Viewing Party
Connect, Experience

Do you have a favorite TV show that will be releasing a new season this fall? Or do you have an old favorite that you'd like to rewatch?

Organize a weekly or biweekly viewing party with some friends. You can host every time, or your group can rotate hosting privileges. This is a great, low-pressure way to connect with others over something you all enjoy.

AUGUST 23
Sit in Awe
Whimsy

Take a moment to reflect on the intricacies of our amazing world. The number of functions your body is doing right at this very moment to support you. The scientific complexities of the environment and how it was created to sustain itself as well as a world of incredible creatures. The interconnectedness of the world and how we all truly depend on one another for food, clothing, transportation, connection, and safety.

Experience the awe of the incredible intricacies of life.

AUGUST 24

GIVE YOURSELF PERMISSION

Fridge and Freezer Deep Clean

Self-Care, Home

Today give yourself permission to deep clean your refrigerator and freezer. Is this an urgent need? No. Will you later be glad that you set aside this time? Absolutely.

After a summer of cookouts, it could surely use a little TLC. Check expiration dates and toss items that have expired or gone bad.

These less glamorous parts of life build the foundation and create room for the more glamorous parts. Your future self will thank you!

AUGUST 25

Go on an *Ísbíltúr*

Whimsy, Experience

The Icelandic tradition of a leisurely drive to go get ice cream is referred to as an *ísbíltúr*, pronounced "ease-beel-tour." The heart of this tradition is to take one's time, take back roads rather than the quickest route, and enjoy the journey.

Take your own ice cream road trip and enjoy the drive!

AUGUST 26

HELLO, LOVER

Heliophile

Whimsy

Heliophile: a lover of the sun

Most people enjoy spending time in the sunshine, and then there are others who really, really love the sun. They're the sun chasers of the world, spending all their time outdoors, or stealing sun breaks as often as they can.

Where are you on the sun-loving spectrum? Are you a true heliophile? Perhaps you could step outside sometime today and soak up some of those rays and see if you fall just a little bit in love with that moment.

AUGUST 27

Write a Review

Experience

Are there any local restaurants, businesses, or places you absolutely love? Your feedback matters! Write them an online review. Your experiences and perspectives will be valued by others as they look into options, and you might just sway someone to check out that place you so enjoy.

AUGUST 28
Color Refresh
Home

Is there a room in your home that has begun to feel a bit stale? The single design tactic that will make the biggest splash is changing the wall color. Play around with new wall color options, and pick out a new paint color or wallpaper pattern to bring new energy into your space.

If you're a renter, chat with your landlord about design options. See if you are allowed to paint with their approval, or look into renter-friendly (easily removable) wallpaper options.

AUGUST 29
Ink Up
Whimsy

While you might not be interested in committing to a permanent tattoo, why not sport some temporary ink to celebrate the end of summer? Pick up some temporary tattoos, and invite a few friends over to join in the fun! There are tons of design options out there for you to choose from, from delicate lines to retro icons.

AUGUST 30
Make a Collage
Create

Depending on where you live, it could be pretty toasty outside by this point in the summer. After months of heat, you may be so over it that you'd like to stay indoors where it's cooler.

Beat the heat by spending some downtime inside collaging. Grab some old magazines, turn on a fun playlist, and let yourself get carried away! Pick a theme for your collage or explore photomontage, and see what themes emerge as you go.

And if you need a little extra help to get started, check out the artwork from some notable collage and photomontage creators such as Pablo Picasso, Man Ray, Henri Matisse, Loui Jover, Georges Braque, Charles Dellschau, Hannah Höch, and Raoul Hausmann.

AUGUST 31

Find Rejuvenation in the Great Outdoors

Nature

In the woods too, a man casts off his years, as the snake his slough, and at what period soever of life, is always a child. In the woods, is perpetual youth.

RALPH WALDO EMERSON

In modern days dominated by screens, we can easily distract ourselves from the wonders that exist outside our own front doors. Reflect on where and how you spent your time last month. Can you recall a specific moment when you stopped to feel the sun on your skin, to close your eyes and let the breeze ruffle your hair? How can you create opportunities to ditch the screens and take in the great gift of nature in the days ahead?

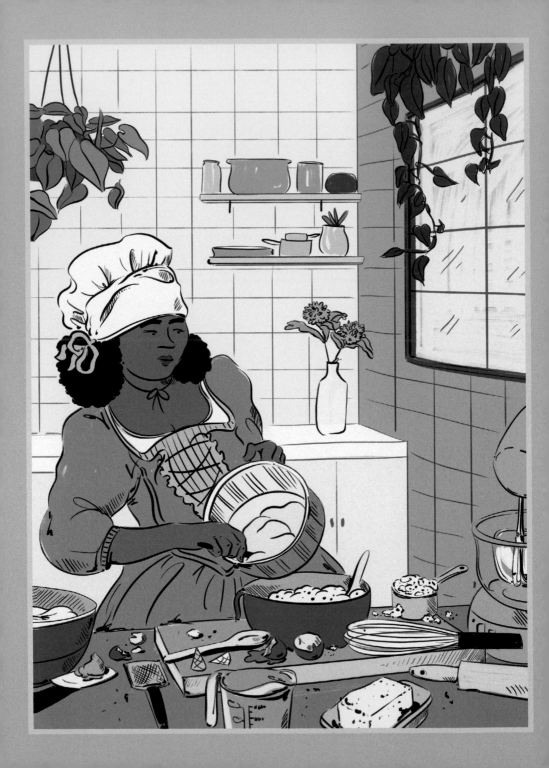

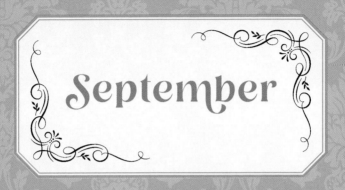

September

SEPTEMBER 1
Find Buoyancy Through Stories
Experience

You can never get a cup of tea large enough or a book
long enough to suit me.

C. S. LEWIS

When was the last time you allowed someone else's words to truly delight you?

What were some of your favorite stories as a child?

What are some books that border on the absurd or that create such fantastical worlds that astound you?

What are some popular blogs that inspire you?

Allow yourself to get carried away through reading words and stories that buoy your spirit.

SEPTEMBER 2
Be As Good As Bread
Identity, Whimsy

───── ITALIAN SAYING OF THE DAY ─────

Buono come il pane
Translation: good as bread

This phrase is used to describe a person with a heart of gold. He or she is somebody who's known for being kind, generous, and trustworthy. You can use the phrase as a blanket description of a good person or as a praise for someone's character. Coming from a culture that reveres its bread the way that Italy does, this is quite a compliment.

Who in your life represents being *buono come il pane*? Take a moment today to tell them. Maybe even treat them to a homemade or artisan loaf with a special note attached to it letting them know just how good they are.

SEPTEMBER 3
Scatter Joy
Nature, Experience

Search your pantry for some cereal, crackers, or seeds you can spare and head outside. Stroll until you find feathered friends—whether in the trees or peacefully paddling across a pond. Gently scatter the morsels you brought, remembering the joy and relief you've experienced when someone in your life showed up at the perfect time with *just* the thing you needed.

Today *you* are the joy scatterer, showing up at just the right time with just the right thing to provide for these beautiful winged creatures.

SEPTEMBER 4
Become a Student Again
Experience

Learning something new can really help to breathe new life into an otherwise repetitive or stagnant schedule.

Sign up for a class to learn a new skill. Cooking, calligraphy, woodworking—whatever strikes your fancy!

SEPTEMBER 5
Auditory Story
Experience, Home

Amid life's demands, it can sometimes be tough to find time to sit down and read. Why not bring a book to accompany you? Select a title you've been wanting to read and check out an audio edition. (Most libraries have audiobooks available to borrow for free!) Listen while you drive, do chores around the house, or cook dinner, and let your mind be transported into a story as you tend to the tasks of your day.

SEPTEMBER 6
Surround Yourself
Connect

Surround yourself with the dreamers, the doers, the believers, and thinkers; but most of all surround yourself with those who see greatness within you even when you don't see it yourself.

EDMUND LEE (ATTRIBUTED)

SEPTEMBER 7
Choose Your September Theme Song
Whimsy

September quickens as summer days fade away and the fall breezes in. Imagine this month as a gust of still-warm air whipped into a breeze against your skin. The crunch of drying grass underfoot and the hint of an autumn not yet fully arrived. Select a September theme song that feels like a promise of something yet to come.

SEPTEMBER 8
Fall Essentials
Self-Care, Identity

Make a list of your current fall essentials. What are your must-haves? Think of that go-to sweater, savory autumn snacks, hangout spots, favorite activities, seasonal movies, or that autumnal playlist.

Poll your friends to see what their lists are, then keep these fall essentials lists in mind as you're planning events together in the weeks to come.

SEPTEMBER 9
Immerse Yourself in Sacred Words
Self-Care

Borrow the sacred words from Saint Francis of Assisi. Allow his inspired wisdom to lift your gaze and reset the way you move through your day.

> Lord, make me an instrument of thy peace.
>
> Where there is hatred, let me sow love,
>
> where there is injury, pardon;
>
> where there is doubt, faith;
>
> where there is despair, hope;
>
> where there is darkness, light;
>
> and where there is sadness, joy.
>
> O Divine Master, grant that I may not so much seek
>
> to be consoled as to console,
>
> to be understood as to understand,
>
> to be loved as to love.
>
> For it is in giving that we receive,
>
> it is in pardoning that we are pardoned,
>
> and it is in dying that we are born to eternal life.
>
> SAINT FRANCIS OF ASSISI

SEPTEMBER 10

Batrachophile

Whimsy

Batrachophile: fondness of amphibians,
such as frogs, newts, and salamanders

Whether you're a real batrachophile or suffer from ranidaphobia, can you find something new to appreciate about our amphibian friends?

SEPTEMBER 11

Thank First Responders

Connect

Look into ways you can support the public safety workers in your community: firefighters, police officers, and emergency medical responders. These jobs have high demands and come with risks to their personal safety. Reach out to your local fire station, and see how you can support them, whether it's dropping off a meal, delivering flowers, or financially supporting a specific need of theirs.

SEPTEMBER 12
Find Your Favorite Hand Soap
Experience

As dull as hand soap may sound, it is something you use every day, multiple times a day, so why not make it a lovely experience? Next time you need a soap refill, explore some new brands and scents. Choose the mood you're wanting to create through the scent experience and let that guide your decision.

Did you know there are many different types of soap? Here are some ideas from around the world to help you delve into the world of soap:

- castile soap
- marseille soap
- aleppo soap
- African black soap
- nabulsi soap
- vegan soap
- *azul e branco* soap
- lava soap
- saltwater soap
- shaving soap

SEPTEMBER 13
Make a Skillet Apple Pie
Create

What is more rustic than making a homemade apple pie in a cast-iron skillet? (Don't worry; you won't need to tell anyone that you used a pre-made piecrust!)

Skillet Apple Pie
Prep time: 1 hour | Cook time: 1 hour | Serves: 6 to 8

Ingredients

2 pounds Granny Smith apples

2 pounds Braeburn apples

1 teaspoon ground cinnamon

3/4 cup granulated sugar, plus 2 tablespoons for topping

1/2 cup salted butter

1 cup firmly packed light brown sugar

2 refrigerated piecrusts

1 egg white

1/2 teaspoon salt

Optional: a sprinkle of sea salt flakes

Instructions

1. Preheat the oven to 350 degrees Fahrenheit. Peel the apples and cut them into $^1/_2$-inch-thick wedges. Toss the apples with the cinnamon and $^3/_4$ cup granulated sugar.

2. Melt the butter in a 10-inch cast-iron skillet over medium heat; add brown sugar and cook, stirring constantly, 1 to 2 minutes, or until the sugar is dissolved. Remove the skillet from the heat, and place one piecrust in the skillet over the brown sugar mixture.

3. Spoon the apple mixture over the piecrust, and top with the second piecrust.

4. Whisk the egg white until foamy. Brush the top of the piecrust with the egg white; sprinkle with 2 tablespoons of granulated sugar and $^1/_2$ teaspoon of salt. Cut four or five slits in the top for the steam to escape.

5. Bake for 1 hour to 1 hour and 10 minutes, or until golden brown and bubbly, covering the pie with aluminum foil during the last 10 minutes to prevent excessive browning.

6. Cool on a wire rack for 30 minutes before serving. Top with sea salt flakes if you want a lovely sweet-and-salty flavor combo.

SEPTEMBER 14
Autumn Affirmations
Self-Care, Identity

It's time for your autumn affirmations! This time of year often has a quickening feeling as days begin to get shorter and schedules get busier. It's easy to become less intentional about the words you speak to yourself as you go from place to place, honoring obligations and taking care of what needs tending.

Spend some time thinking about the words you need to hear during this upcoming season, and write down five affirmations, truths, prayers, or hopes. Place the list somewhere you'll see it every day: on your bathroom mirror, next to your coffee maker, in the laundry room, or inside your planner.

Here are a few to help get you started:

- As the seasons change, I embrace the new changes in my life.
- I will prioritize rest and recovery.
- Everything happens at just the right time.
- I am thankful for each new day.
- Every day is a new beginning.
- I am open to experiencing just how good life gets for me today.

SEPTEMBER 15

RECALIBRATE YOUR MORNING ROUTINE

Make Your Own Honey-Do List

Self-Care

Taking time to make lists can have a dramatic effect on your well-being, including helping memory and improving focus.[20]

Whether you write it in the morning or review a list you've created the night before, taking just a few minutes to map out your daily to-do list will help you intentionally organize your time, energy, and attention so you can approach your days with purpose.

Don't neglect the often forgotten—but just as vital—niceties in the midst of your daily responsibilities, like smiling at a stranger or taking a deep breath in and exhaling slowly. Especially when our schedules are demanding, we need to remind ourselves to do these little things that can affect our days in big ways.

Remember: your time is precious, and you owe it to yourself to use it well.

SEPTEMBER 16

Enjoy Anonymity

Experience

> If fame belonged to me, I could not escape her—if she
> did not, the longest day would pass me on the chase—
> and the approbation of my dog would forsake me then.
> My barefoot rank is better.
>
> EMILY DICKINSON

It's easy to idealize a life in the spotlight—the fame, the glamour, the privileges it brings. But these things come at a price. What a joy it is to live without constant attention—and constant scrutiny—and to savor the deeply felt joys of life's most precious gifts. Today revel in being the leading lady of your own story, where your contentment and quality of life are not subject to public opinion.

SEPTEMBER 17
Host a Block Party
Connect

Now that the temperatures are beginning to cool and families are back from summer travels, it's the perfect time to get neighbors together for a little block party! Send out invites, encourage people to bring a snack or drink to share, and find some games or a firepit to set up. Some neighborhoods allow you to block off the street for an evening if you get a permit ahead of time, so do some investigating and decide what works best for the place where you live.

It's easy to get wrapped up in the busyness of individual schedules, but what a great opportunity to reconnect with the people in your own backyard.

SEPTEMBER 18

BECOME A FINANCE QUEEN

Diversify Revenue Streams

Self-Care

If you're not fluent in the finance world, you may hear the phrase "diversify revenue streams" and think, *Um, what?* Diversifying revenue streams means getting paid from a variety of sources. This includes full-time work, part-time jobs, side gigs, rental properties, and investments.

If you're feeling a bit tight in the finance department and a pay raise at your main gig isn't in your near future, look into how you can begin to diversify your income streams, whether it's now or down the road.

SEPTEMBER 19

Find Your Autumn Scent

Beauty, Identity

Is there anything better than the first smells of fall? Welcome this cozy season by finding your signature autumn scent. Look for sweets and spices like cinnamon, pumpkin, apple, chai, sandalwood, brown sugar, vanilla, nutmeg, and smoky campfire.

SEPTEMBER 20
Set an Intention for Your Legacy
Identity

What kind of legacy do you want to leave behind? An influence on your family, your community, an industry, or an entire cultural norm? Reflect on some areas where you want to make an impact, and brainstorm up to three steps you can take to begin building your lasting legacy today.

SEPTEMBER 21
Take What You Need
Whimsy, Self-Care

Take what you need, and carry it with you for the rest of your day:

- motivation to truly listen to someone who has an opinion that differs from your own
- motivation to compliment an acquaintance or stranger
- motivation to open up in a conversation, sharing an experience to grow closer to another person
- motivation to extend forgiveness to someone who has unintentionally hurt you

SEPTEMBER 22

HELLO, LOVER

Oenophile

Whimsy

Oenophile: a connoisseur of wine, a person who loves tasting wines

Are you a connoisseur of wine? Or perhaps coffee, tea, or a particular cuisine? What could you become a connoisseur of?

SEPTEMBER 23

Create Your Own Awards

Whimsy, Connect

Doesn't it feel great to be recognized every now and then? And doesn't it feel even better when you are recognized unexpectedly?

Create your own awards for your teammates at work, friends, or family. Get crafty by making them yourself, or keep it simple and print out some templates, which you can find online.

Hand out these awards to recognize people for their character, quirks, or contributions. They will, without a doubt, bring a spark of joy to their day!

SEPTEMBER 24
Discover Your Spirit Animal
Whimsy, Identity

What animal best embodies you? Consider your energy, your skills, and the ways you interact with the world. An animated and curious cockatoo? A gangly yet strong moose? Brainstorm and think of what animal you most identify with and why.

SEPTEMBER 25
A Lucky Find
Whimsy

———— FRENCH WORD OF THE DAY ————

Trouvaille
Translation: a valuable discovery or lucky find; something nice discovered by chance

What was your last lucky find?

SEPTEMBER 26
Home Edit
Home

Your own taste and love, if you set about the work in the right spirit, will teach you better than anyone else can do. Arrange the necessary articles and all the embellishments with care and thought, so that when you stand at the door and survey the work, the room shall lie before you like a picture, speaking of cheerfulness, rest, and comfort.

H. W. BEECHER, *Motherly Talks with Young Housekeepers*

Which decorative items in your home are out of sync with the feeling you want to create? Are those eclectic photo frames detracting from the clean, streamlined look you want in your home now? Are those minimalistic lamps throwing off the English-cottage vibe you're desiring?

Go room by room and take note of the items that you may want to swap out or refresh. Check out local estate sales, online marketplaces, and consignment shops to help you achieve the style you are dreaming of!

SEPTEMBER 27
Create a Spa Experience at Home
Home, Self-Care

You can create a luxurious and relaxing spa-like experience by hanging a bunch of beautiful eucalyptus leaves in your shower at home.

Simply gather branches, clear the leaves from the bottom of the stems, and tie them tightly together with a long piece of string or twine around the stem bottoms. Use the ends of the string to hang the bunch from your showerhead or a hook secured to the shower wall. Be careful not to position the bouquet directly under the water stream. The undiluted eucalyptus oil might irritate your skin, so allow the steam from your shower to activate and release the oils into the air while the eucalyptus itself stays relatively dry.

And if fresh eucalyptus isn't available near you, no worries; try adding some eucalyptus essential oil to a diffuser for the same effect.

SEPTEMBER 28
Go Apple Picking
Experience, Connect

Head out to a local apple orchard, and pick your own apples. It's a great way to experience the bounty of the fall harvest firsthand.

SEPTEMBER 29
GIVE YOURSELF PERMISSION
Make Those Doctor's Appointments
Self-Care

This is the perfect time to give yourself permission to prioritize scheduling those routine medical appointments that may have fallen off your radar—before all the fall and winter holiday festivities begin.

Whether it's the dentist, dermatologist, eye doctor, or your primary care provider, double-check your calendar to make sure you've got those appointments scheduled, especially before the next calendar year rolls around.

Your physical health is an absolute priority; don't let it fall by the wayside!

SEPTEMBER 30

Replenish Your Energy with a Bit of Comfort

Coziness

As the lazy days of summer fade to fall, the quickened rhythm of this season can make the hours fly by in a flurry of tasks to be done.

Have you started to feel worn down or even exhausted by the pace of things? Great satisfaction can be found in fulfilling our responsibilities well, but we mustn't let our days become a series of chores and checked boxes.

What ways have you been able to find comfort—even in the fleeting moments and smallest ways—that make you feel replenished? We can't always spend an entire day at a spa being pampered, but we *can* bring intention to the little moments each day. What can you do for yourself today—and in the days following—to find a bit of rest and restoration?

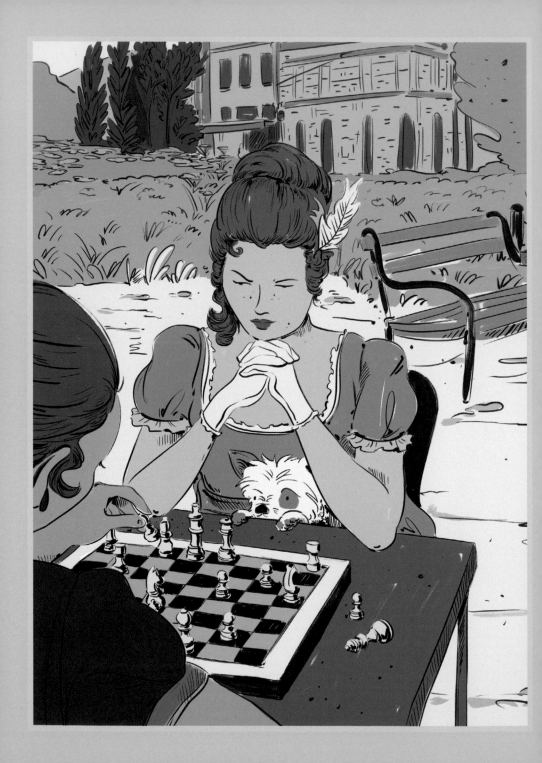

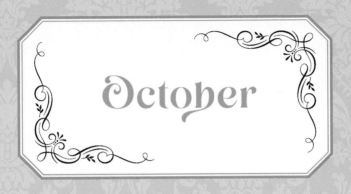

October

OCTOBER 1
Host an Autumn Drink Tasting
Experience

I'm so glad I live in a world where there are Octobers.

L. M. MONTGOMERY, *Anne of Green Gables*

October is the beginning for all things cozy. And what's more cozy than warm beverages?

Coordinate an autumn drink-tasting party with your friends. It can be for anything you like: mulled wine, coffee, cocoa, hot toddies, or warm apple cider! After selecting the drink, have each guest bring a different variation or brand of that drink. Line them up and do a side-by-side tasting, comparing flavor notes, textures, and anything that makes sense for that specific drink.

If you want to go the extra mile, look up tasting charts for the sampling item, and use them at the party for everyone to reference. They may help you identify flavors that you hadn't noticed before, and you'll be able to call upon your newly acquired knowledge the next time that drink is served!

OCTOBER 2
Create an Autumn Tablescape
Home, Create

Create an elevated autumnal tablescape. Look up inspiration pics to work from, or go with your instincts!

Incorporate a few elements that are guaranteed to elevate your dining experience: place mats and chargers, candle votives or tall candlesticks, dried seasonal grasses and flowers, and harvested items like pumpkins, gourds, apples, or pomegranates.

OCTOBER 3
Reflect on Your Proud Moments
Identity

Take a few moments to journal about the moments, decisions, and actions you've taken that you're most proud of. Reach back into the archives of your memory, and think of examples that stand out from years ago. Next, focus on more recent memories. Are there any current opportunities that you want to act on to make your future self proud?

OCTOBER 4
Nourish Yourself with Stuffed Acorn Squash
Create

This cozy meal full of delicious, nutrient-dense fall ingredients will leave you feeling nourished—perfect for a crisp autumn day.

Stuffed Acorn Squash

Prep time: 20 minutes | Cook time: 45 minutes | Serves: 4

Ingredients

2 medium acorn squash

2 tablespoons extra-virgin olive oil, divided

$1/2$ teaspoon fine sea salt, divided

$1/2$ cup quinoa, rinsed

1 cup water

1 cup chickpeas, rinsed and drained

$1/4$ cup dried cranberries

$1/4$ cup raw pepitas (hulled pumpkin seeds)

$1/4$ cup chopped green onion

$1/4$ cup chopped fresh flat-leaf parsley, plus 1 tablespoon for garnish

1 clove garlic, pressed or minced

1 tablespoon lemon juice

$3/4$ cup grated Parmesan cheese

$1/2$ cup crumbled goat cheese or feta

Instructions

1. Preheat the oven to 400 degrees Fahrenheit, and line a large, rimmed baking sheet with parchment paper for easy cleanup.

2. To prepare the squash, use a sharp chef's knife to slice through it from the tip to the stem: pierce the squash in the center along a depression line, then cut through the tip, and finish by slicing through the top portion just next to the stem. Use a large spoon to scoop out the seeds and stringy bits inside, and discard those pieces.

3. Place the squash halves, cut-side up, on the parchment-lined pan. Drizzle 1 tablespoon of the olive oil over the squash, and sprinkle with $1/4$ teaspoon of the salt. Rub the oil into the cut sides of the squash, then turn them over so the cut sides are facedown in the pan. Bake until the squash flesh is easily pierced through by a fork, about 30 to 45 minutes. Leave the oven on.

4. Meanwhile, cook the quinoa. In a medium saucepan, combine the rinsed quinoa and water. Bring the mixture to a boil over medium-high heat, then reduce the heat as necessary to maintain a gentle simmer. Simmer, uncovered, until all the water is absorbed, 12 to 18 minutes. Remove the pot from the heat, and stir in the chickpeas and cranberries. Cover, and let the mixture steam for 5 minutes. Uncover and fluff the quinoa with a fork.

5. In a medium skillet, toast the pepitas over medium heat, stirring frequently, until the pepitas are turning golden on the edges and making little popping noises, about 4 to 5 minutes. Set aside.

6. Pour the fluffed quinoa mixture into a medium-sized bowl. Add the toasted pepitas, green onion, parsley, garlic, lemon juice, the remaining $1/4$ teaspoon salt, and the remaining 1 tablespoon olive oil. Stir until the ingredients are evenly distributed. Taste and add additional salt, if necessary.

7. If the mixture is very hot, let it cool for a few minutes before adding the Parmesan cheese and goat cheese. Gently stir the mixture to combine.

8. Turn the cooked squash halves over so the cut sides are facing up. Divide the quinoa mixture evenly between the squash halves with a large spoon. Return the squash to the oven, and bake for 15 to 18 minutes, until the cheesy quinoa is golden.

9. Garnish the stuffed squash with the remaining tablespoon of chopped parsley, and serve warm.

OCTOBER 5
Take the Scenic Route
Whimsy, Beauty

Rather than taking the most efficient route to work, school, or errands, try taking a more scenic path. Wind through neighborhoods, take the back roads, drive past a beautiful overlook. Slow down and soak in the sights that have been waiting patiently for you.

OCTOBER 6
Essential Expectations Only
Self-Care, Whimsy

Between managing all your responsibilities and navigating the constant noise of the modern world, it can begin to feel like you'll never be able to measure up to all that's expected of you. Let go of demands—especially the ones you put on yourself—and spend the day focused on these simple words: today the only things you need to be are silly, honest, and kind.

OCTOBER 7
Choose Your October Theme Song
Whimsy

> October is the month for painted leaves. Their rich glow
> now flashes round the world. As fruits and leaves and
> the day itself acquire a bright tint just before they fall, so
> the year near its setting.

HENRY DAVID THOREAU, *Excursions*

Cool days, cozy nights. Leaves turning red, orange, and brilliant marigold. Plaid shirts and pumpkin spice near the warmth of a fire. Choose an October theme song that feels like these things.

OCTOBER 8
HELLO, LOVER
Bibliophile
Whimsy

Bibliophile: a person with a great fondness of books; a book lover

This would be a great time to gather your fall and winter reading list together for those cozy nights!

OCTOBER 9

Have a Cozy Movie Night

Coziness

Pick a favorite fall film, change into your comfiest clothes, and have yourself a cozy movie night in. Crack open the window to allow the crisp fall air in, and light some candles to add a warm glow to your movie experience. As simple as it is, this may be exactly what you need to recharge your batteries.

OCTOBER 10

Go to a Classic Car Show

Experience

Step back into yesteryear, and go to a classic car show. Note how much changes from decade to decade. Chat with some of the owners, and learn about their care for the cars: what upkeep they do, what restoration projects they've completed, and what got them interested in classic cars.

OCTOBER 11
Ghost a Neighbor
Connect

Take part in the Halloween tradition of "ghosting." Far from the term's new connotation, this type of ghosting involves surprising friends by ding-dong-ditching them and leaving a basket of treats at their door. Gather up a bag of snacks, write a note, and ghost away!

OCTOBER 12
Embrace Quiet
Identity

Whoever you are, bear in mind that appearance is not reality. Some people act like extroverts, but the effort costs them in energy, authenticity, and even physical health. Others seem aloof or self-contained, but their inner landscapes are rich and full of drama. So the next time you see a person with a composed face and a soft voice, remember that inside her mind she might be solving an equation, composing a sonnet, designing a hat. She might, that is, be deploying the powers of quiet.

SUSAN CAIN, *Quiet*

OCTOBER 13
Write a Haiku
Create

I write, erase, rewrite
Erase again, and then
A poppy blooms.

KATSUSHIKA HOKUSAI, "A Poppy Blooms"

A haiku is a type of short form Japanese poetry. Traditional Japanese haiku consist of three phrases that contain a 5–7–5 syllable pattern.

Try your hand at writing a haiku about one small moment in your day in which you found deep contentment. Perhaps it was that first steaming sip of coffee as the sun rose outside the window in the morning or a familiar embrace from a loved one when you returned home at the end of the day.

If you'd like some inspiration, look into the haiku poetry of Ezra Pound, Jack Kerouac, Gary Snyder, and Marlene Mountain.

OCTOBER 14
Saying No So You Can Say Yes
Whimsy

—————— FRENCH PHRASE OF THE DAY ——————

Avoir le beurre et l'argent du beurre
Translation: to have the butter and the butter money

As we say in English, you can't have your cake and eat it too . . . and as the French would say, you can't have the butter and the money you use to buy the butter.

Life is full of compromises, and not bad ones! Choosing where to devote one's time, energy, money, or appetite requires saying yes to something and no to something else.

Reflect on an area of your life in which you've been trying to have the butter and also the butter money. It's likely been causing some strain on your schedule, finances, relationships, or attention. What do you need to say no to right now so you can say a committed and hearty yes to something else? If you're feeling stuck, reflect on what you want your top priorities to be right now, and let that guide your decision.

OCTOBER 15

Outfit Planning

Self-Care

How many times have you been late because you couldn't figure out what to wear? Instead of sifting through your wardrobe with bleary morning eyes or frantically trying on countless clothing combinations, try selecting and setting aside your next day's outfit the night before. Not only will this make your morning go more smoothly, but it will also allow time to spot wrinkles that need tending and avoid any last-minute style blunders that you wouldn't catch in the rush to get out the door.

Set aside a specific place to lay out or hang your outfit for the next day. As you look at your carefully selected outfit, ready for your wear, it will help you envision the day ahead with calmness and optimistic anticipation.

OCTOBER 16
Celebrate Self-Awareness
Self-Care

Cultivating self-awareness can not only help you gain more insights into yourself, but according to *The Washington Post*, it can improve relationships.[21] And according to psychologist Rick Hanson in the same article, this is the key to a life well lived.

As you think about your own life, what's working? What's not working as well as you would like? This awareness is perhaps the first step toward changing patterns and creating a life you love.

OCTOBER 17
Decorate Jack-O'-Lanterns
Whimsy, Create, Connect

Whether you wish to carve, paint, or collage on pumpkins, invite some friends over to decorate jack-o'-lanterns.

OCTOBER 18
Play a Board Game in the Park
Whimsy, Connect

There's something so "New York–in-the-fall" about older gentlemen playing chess in the park on a crisp autumn morning. Bundled in their jackets, steaming coffee at their sides. Strategizing and spearing one another with friendly jokes.

Whether it's a game of chess, mancala, or Scrabble, invite a friend to head to the park for a morning match!

OCTOBER 19
Expand Your Definition of *Romanticize*
Whimsy

In the opening epigraph, we included a quote by Novalis on romanticizing the world (see page vi). To help you cultivate your sense of self-awareness and deepen your love affair with your life, how have you become more aware of the magic, mystery, and wonder of the world?

OCTOBER 20
Learn About Diwali, the Festival of Lights
Experience

Diwali is one of India's most widely celebrated holidays of the year. Celebrating the victory of light over darkness, or good over evil, the festival gets its name from the Sanskrit word *dipavali*, meaning "row of lights." The festival lasts for five days and is celebrated during the Hindu lunisolar month Karttika, which falls in late October or early November.[22]

Each day of the festival holds its own significance. Because Diwali is celebrated by a diverse range of people from varying faith backgrounds and cultural traditions, many people celebrate the holiday in their own unique ways. According to an article in *Good Housekeeping*, this is generally a time for family gatherings, performing acts of *dana* (charitable giving) and *seva* (selfless service), deep cleaning and decorating the home, performing religious ceremonies, stringing up lights, and reflecting on deeply held values.[23]

Look into Diwali celebrations in your area. Connect with those who celebrate, and learn more about what this holiday means to them.

OCTOBER 21
Take What You Need
Whimsy, Self-Care

As seasons change, so do our needs. And sometimes as things change, we need a little extra boost to get us through.

Take what you need, and carry it with you for the rest of your day:

- belief that a win will come your way
- confidence that if something doesn't work out, you aren't the problem; it's just not the right fit
- patience to let things unfold as they need to
- perseverance to keep going when things are challenging and mundane
- permission to walk away from something you've outgrown
- faith that everything will work out for the best
- creativity to come up with fresh ideas
- optimism to go into your day looking for the best outcome

OCTOBER 22

Uncover Your Personal Style Roots

Great personal style is an extreme curiosity about yourself.

IRIS APFEL, interior designer and fashion icon

Is there a clothing item or accessory that you've been itching to try on but feels too far out of your style comfort zone? Or maybe a bold new color or pattern? Why not get curious?

Just go for it, and see how wearing a new style makes you feel. Discover how it affects the way you carry yourself throughout your day.

Or visit some clothing boutiques or clothing departments that you've never been to. See how wearing a new style can maybe give you a fresh perspective and help you define a style that's more authentically you.

OCTOBER 23

Sights and Sounds of Autumn

Self-Care, Nature

Go for an afternoon walk and leave the headphones at home. Listen to the crunch of fall leaves underfoot. Notice the changing trees as they take on autumn's gold and rust hues. What a gift the changing seasons give us: with each new era, we get to meet ourselves all over again.

OCTOBER 24

Add a New Soup to Your Repertoire

Create

Soup can be dressed up or down and makes you feel great no matter the occasion. Try a new recipe to add to your go-to meals this season!

Here are a few you may want to try:

- Italian: Italian wedding soup
- West African: peanut soup
- Thai: coconut chickpea curry soup
- Mexican: green chicken enchilada soup
- French: wild mushroom chowder with bacon and leeks

OCTOBER 25

HELLO, LOVER

Selenophile

Whimsy

Selenophile: a person who loves the moon

Some barely notice the moon while others set their calendars by it. Some selenophiles love the moon so much they perform monthly rituals and ceremonies as a way to say goodbye to the old things that no longer serve them and hello to the new opportunities that await. During the next full moon or new moon, set your intentions for what you'd like to call in during the next moon cycle.

OCTOBER 26

Start a Puzzle

Whimsy, Connect

Start a puzzle in a public space. Maybe at your desk at work, on your front porch, or on a picnic table at the park. Invite passersby to join in and help find the pieces for a few places. See what conversations it sparks! Leave it out for a few days and see who stops by to keep puzzling.

OCTOBER 27

Cozy Connection

Whimsy, Home, Coziness, Connect, Self-Care

--------- NORWEGIAN WORD OF THE DAY ---------

Koselig: a feeling of deep contentment, provided by a person, place, or atmosphere; experiencing happiness and personal well-being through a combination of nature, companionship, and coziness

May you experience a deep sense of *koselig* as you go about your day today.

OCTOBER 28

Embrace the Small Steps

Dream, Self-Care

Has the overwhelming nature of a big dream or goal been keeping you from getting started? Put the end goal to the side, and focus only on the very first step you need to take to begin the journey.

OCTOBER 29
Go Puddle Jumping
Whimsy

Remember that childhood love of jumping in puddles after a big rainstorm? Well, why not enjoy a little puddle jumping now? After the next shower, jump into your rain boots and go for a stroll. Enjoy the childlike joy when you make an extra-big splash.

OCTOBER 30
Host a Pet Costume Contest
Whimsy, Connect

While some people don't love dressing up, who can resist adorable pets in costume? Host a neighborhood pet parade. Invite families to bring their dogs, cats, guinea pigs, or any non-human members of their family to join! For the less portable or less social pets, have the owners snap a picture at home and submit it to the judges.

OCTOBER 31

Celebrate Who You Are As a Main Character

Identity

Developing a mindset and behavior pattern tuned toward your own self-improvement is undoubtedly a healthy practice, but we mustn't let a focus on bettering ourselves distract us from the goodness that's already there. Step outside of yourself for a moment and examine what makes you *you*.

What do you like about yourself?

What do you find admirable or endearing?

What are the unique gifts that you offer the world?

How do you better the lives of those around you?

Going forward, try to develop a habit of looking at yourself with a little more kindness and appreciation.

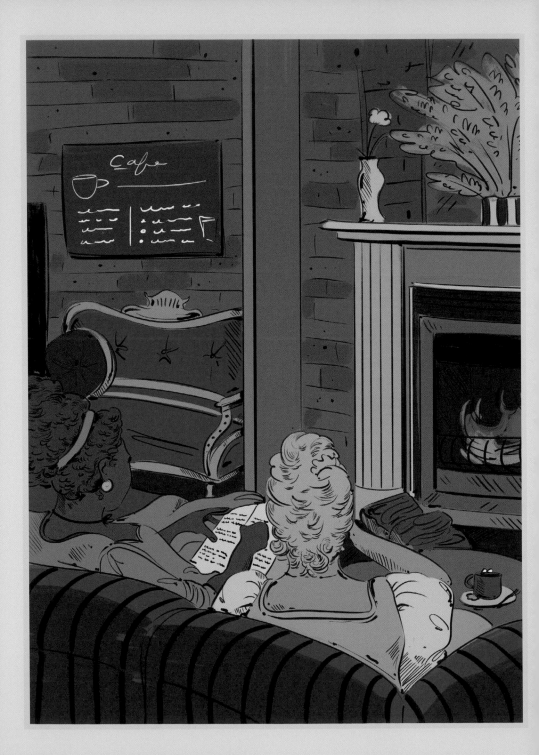

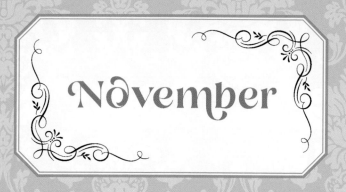

November

NOVEMBER 1
Send a Postcard
Connect

Who doesn't love to receive snail mail? Pick up a postcard from a local shop, or better yet, create your own! Send it to a friend with a quick note to let them know you're thinking of them.

NOVEMBER 2
Go on a Historic Architecture Tour
Experience

Wherever you live, big city or small town, there is bound to be a historical building nearby that offers tours. Old theaters, churches, courthouses, train stations, estates—these historic spaces are dripping with symbolism and craftsmanship of years past and the kinds of beauty that aren't featured in modern buildings. Sign up for a tour and get acquainted with a local architectural treasure—and just maybe fall a little more in love with your city.

NOVEMBER 3
Preserve Your Family's Stories Through Food
Create, Connect

Perhaps the most precious heirlooms are family recipes.
Like a physical heirloom, they remind us from whom
and where we came and give others, in a bite, the story
of another people from another place and another time.
Yet unlike a lost physical heirloom, recipes are a part of
our history that can be re-created over and over again.

STANLEY TUCCI, *Taste: My Life Through Food*

As Stanley noted in his food memoir, family recipes might just be the most precious family heirloom of all, with their ability to be re-created for years to come, telling the story of those who came before you.

If you don't already have your beloved family recipes written down, reach out to the family members who have them. Save them and continue to share them. And when you do serve those special meals, share the stories that come along with them, transporting your guests to the time and place from which those recipes came.

NOVEMBER 4
Create an Autumn Flat Lay
Create, Nature, Beauty

Head outside to your fall palette of jewel-tone leaves, seeds, and dried foliage. Gather whatever natural materials catch your eye, and lay them out in an artistic flat lay—the same kind of visually appealing design from a bird's-eye view that you created in the spring (see April 13)—on the ground for passersby to enjoy.

Look up nature flat lays beforehand if you need some inspiration!

NOVEMBER 5
HELLO, LOVER
Dendrophile
Whimsy

Dendrophile: a person who loves forests and trees

If you're not already a certified dendrophile, have you considered forest bathing? The idea of *shinrin-yoku*—taking in the forest atmosphere—emerged from Japan,[24] and is believed to be an antidote to burnout. If you haven't done so lately, take a walk in the woods or a nearby park today.

NOVEMBER 6

Cultivate Ambience

Home, Coziness

Never underestimate the flickering glow of candlelight. Its warm, gentle light and subtle sounds are perfect for bringing you into the present moment as you admire the candle's beauty and ease into a slower state of mind.

Take a quick stroll around your home, and see what nooks and surfaces you could use to cultivate ambience to help you wind down in the evenings. Your bathroom counter, the coffee table in the living room, the dresser in your bedroom. Stock up on candlesticks, tealights, and a few new candleholders to have on hand this winter.

NOVEMBER 7

Choose Your November Theme Song

Whimsy

Sweet November has arrived, and with it, all its comforts. This month choose a nostalgic theme song that feels like home—one that you can imagine playing in the background of a treasured memory or one that captures the emotions of a present moment that you'd like to remember.

NOVEMBER 8
Spice Up Your Coffee
Create

Enjoy the taste of the season by adding a cinnamon stick to your morning coffee or tea. This sweet little spice has antioxidants and valuable vitamins and nutrients, but stirring your coffee with a cinnamon stick is also just plain fun.

NOVEMBER 9
Enjoy Some Brussels
Create

Brussels sprouts get a bad rap, but when prepared with the proper seasonings, they are absolutely delectable. These veggies are abundant in the fall and are packed with vitamin C and vitamin K!

The recipe for Dijon Roasted Brussels Sprouts on the following page is a delicious way to work in this seasonal vegetable to your meals.

Dijon Roasted Brussels Sprouts

Prep time: 15 minutes | Cook time: 25 minutes | Serves: 6

Ingredients

$1^1/_2$ pounds brussels sprouts, trimmed and halved

2 tablespoons olive oil

1 tablespoon Dijon mustard

$^1/_2$ teaspoon smoked paprika

$^1/_8$ teaspoon garlic powder

$^1/_8$ teaspoon onion powder

$^1/_2$ teaspoon salt, or to taste

$^1/_4$ teaspoon pepper, or to taste

Instructions

1. Heat the oven to 425 degrees Fahrenheit. Place halved brussels sprouts on a rimmed baking sheet.
2. In a small bowl, whisk the olive oil, mustard, paprika, garlic powder, and onion powder. Pour the seasoning mixture over the veggies, and toss to coat. Spread the brussels sprouts in a single layer, cut-side down, on the baking sheet. Sprinkle with salt.
3. Roast 20 to 30 minutes, or until fork-tender. Sprinkle with pepper, and enjoy the veggies that you never knew could be so delicious!

NOVEMBER 10
Find Your Leaf
Nature, Beauty

Take a few moments today to go on a walk, and be on the lookout for one thing: a beautiful autumn leaf. Bring it home and place the leaf somewhere that you can admire it during the next few days. Think about all the growth it's been through over the past year—from just a bud to a jewel-tone treasure. As the days became shorter, more and more of its true colors shone through.

Here's an excerpt from *Excursions* by Henry David Thoreau to inspire you:

> I formerly thought that it would be worth the while to get a specimen leaf from each changing tree . . . when it had acquired its brightest characteristic color, in its transition from the green to the brown state, outline it, and copy its color exactly, with paint in a book . . . beginning with the earliest reddening—Woodbine and the lake of radical leaves, and coming down through the Maples, Hickories, and Sumachs, and many beautifully freckled leaves less generally known, to the latest Oaks and Aspens. What a memento such a book would be! You would need only to turn over its leaves to take a ramble through the autumn woods whenever you pleased. Or if I could preserve the leaves themselves, unfaded, it would be better still.

NOVEMBER 11
Created to Love and Be Loved
Identity

We must know that we have been created for greater
things, not just to be a number in the world, not just to go
for diplomas and degrees, this work and that work. We
have been created in order to love and to be loved.

SAINT TERESA OF CALCUTTA (ATTRIBUTED)

Saint Teresa of Calcutta—better known as Mother Teresa—knew at the
age of twelve that she was called to be a missionary. She left her parental
home at the age of eighteen and joined the Sisters of Loretto, an Irish
community of nuns with missions in India. She was particularly struck
by witnessing suffering and poverty, and dedicated her entire life to
working among the poorest populations, particularly in the slums of
Calcutta.

In 1950 Mother Teresa founded the Missionaries of Charity, whose
main goal was to love and tend to the needs of the poorest and most
destitute people in India. Today the Catholic charity continues to care
for sick and impoverished populations all over the world.[25]

Mother Teresa often spoke of doing small things with great love.
How does her legacy inspire you to let go of worries about personal acco-
lades and achievements and instead make some small effort—one done
with great love—to tend to the needs of those around you?

NOVEMBER 12
Choose Your Alter Ego for a Day
Whimsy, Identity

The play's the thing
Wherein I'll catch the conscience of the king.

WILLIAM SHAKESPEARE, *Hamlet*

Have you ever watched a film, attended a play, or read a book and instantly connected with one of the characters? So much so that part of you wished you could be that person? Perhaps you were drawn to their buoyancy in the face of challenges, their wit, their humor, their ingenuity, their elegance, their kindness, their intelligence, their tenacity and grit, or maybe their devotion to a cause.

Brainstorm a list of the fictional characters you've most admired throughout your life and jot them down in your journal.

Then select one of the characters—and characteristics—you would like to embody today. As you go throughout your day, imagine what they would be thinking about and how they would act, and let that guide you.

NOVEMBER 13
Every Leaf Is a Flower
Nature

Autumn [is] a second spring when every leaf is a flower.

ALBERT CAMUS, *The Misunderstanding*

Faux or fresh, gather together an autumn bouquet of leaves and pumpkins to display in your home or office.

NOVEMBER 14
Redefine Strength
Whimsy

"Who do you think are the strongest?" asked the boy.

"The soft hearted and the honest" said the horse.

"The ones who can resist cake" said the mole.

CHARLIE MACKESY, *The Boy, the Mole, the Fox, and the Horse*

Take a moment today to notice and celebrate your many strengths and be sure to put them to use in ways that nourish your soul.

NOVEMBER 15

RECALIBRATE YOUR MORNING ROUTINE

Get a Good Night's Sleep

Self-Care

The most impactful thing you can do for your morning begins the night before. Getting a good night's sleep is imperative to your overall health, and you can adopt a few simple habits to help you wind down from the day. Avoid caffeine and strenuous activity close to your ideal bedtime, and swap out the late-night screen time for the pages of a book instead. Taking a warm bath or shower in the evening can also help alleviate the day's stress and beckon you forth to a relaxing night's rest. Make your bedroom into a sanctuary with fresh bed linens, soft lamp lighting, and relaxing essential oils in scents like chamomile, bergamot, sandalwood, or lavender.

Create an evening ritual that will help you ease into sleep and greet the next day feeling rested, rejuvenated, and hopeful for what's ahead.

NOVEMBER 16

Find Joy in Self-Forgetfulness

Whimsy, Nature, Experience, Connect

Joy tends to involve some transcendence of self. It's when the skin barrier between you and some other person or entity fades away and you feel fused together. Joy is present when mother and baby are gazing adoringly into each other's eyes, when a hiker is overwhelmed by beauty in the woods and feels at one with nature, when a gaggle of friends are dancing deliriously in unison. . . . Joy often involves self-forgetting.

DAVID BROOKS, *The Second Mountain: The Quest for a Moral Life*

NOVEMBER 17

Cheers

Whimsy

—————— NORWEGIAN WORD OF THE DAY ——————

Skål: a Scandinavian toast of friendship and goodwill that can be offered when drinking, sharing a meal, or sitting down to a formal event

NOVEMBER 18

Find a Fireside Nook

Coziness, Experience, Connect

As temperatures dip, there is nothing quite as cozy as spending time by the fire. Look up restaurants or coffee shops with fireplaces in your area. Invite a friend and enjoy an afternoon or evening by the crackling glow!

NOVEMBER 19

HELLO, LOVER

Chionophile

Whimsy

Chionophile: a person who thrives in cold weather

The cold weather can be exhilarating! Tap into your inner chionophile and take a chilly walk in the woods, experiment with ice baths, or even prepare yourself for a polar bear plunge in a local body of water.

NOVEMBER 20

Listen to the Music

Whimsy, Experience

Turn on a song you've been loving lately, and really pay attention to the lyrics. What appeals to you about the song? The message, the melody, the instruments? Savor the song by turning it on repeat a few times, enjoying not only the experience itself but also a deeper understanding of why you're drawn to it.

NOVEMBER 21

Take What You Need

Whimsy, Self-Care

Take what you need, and carry it with you for the rest of your day:

- groundedness
- focus
- laughter
- ingenuity
- spunk

NOVEMBER 22
Practice Gratitude for Friends
Self-Care, Identity

This time of year is marked by thankfulness, counting blessings, and acknowledging the goodness in life. Take a few moments to journal about the friends, acquaintances, or mentors you are most grateful for. Jot down their names and either a few characteristics that capture them or specific memories with them that you hold dear.

NOVEMBER 23
Practice Gratitude for Places
Self-Care, Identity

Spend some time today to journal about the places you are most grateful for. These could be nostalgic places you visited during childhood, places from your faraway travels, or places that have more recently become meaningful to you. If one of these spots is nearby, do this exercise in the very place that you hold so dear.

NOVEMBER 24
Practice Gratitude for Family
Self-Care, Identity

> Happy families are all alike; every unhappy family is
> unhappy in its own way.
>
> LEO TOLSTOY, *Anna Karenina*

During this season we often spend time with family, which can bring
out the best in us—and sometimes the worst. As well as we know our
families, it can be easy to get into the cycle of focusing on the frustrating
dynamics.

While it's worth acknowledging and addressing anything that
impedes good communication and bonding, it's just as important (if not
more so) to reflect on aspects of family dynamics and your upbringing
that you are grateful for.

What memories do you cherish?

What positive qualities did your family teach you?

Write these down and consider sharing them with your family
members.

NOVEMBER 25
Practice Gratitude for Decisions
Self-Care, Identity

Making major life decisions, especially as we grow older and have more responsibilities to take into consideration, is challenging, to say the least. Choices can feel paralyzing or invigorating at different turns.

Consider some of the positive decisions you've made in the past year. These could be decisions you made to change the way you were spending your time, choosing to pursue a new career opportunity, setting new boundaries for your well-being, or maybe even intentionally savoring the everyday by romanticizing your life.

What decisions from the past year are you grateful for? Whether big or small, they are all worth celebrating.

NOVEMBER 26

Practice Gratitude for Personal Growth

Self-Care, Identity

Reflect on the ways you've grown in the past ten years—emotionally, relationally, mentally, and physically.

Have you improved your planning skills? Are you better at not taking yourself too seriously? Have you improved your self-care in a certain area? Have you grown in awareness for others' needs? Jot down a list of ways you've grown and savor it for a few moments. Some of these are things only you will ever know that have shifted the way you experience your everyday, making you an even brighter and fuller version of yourself. And that, friend, is a beautiful thing.

For inspiration, reflect on these words from *Character Building* by Booker T. Washington:

> I want you to resolve that you are going to put into this year the hardest and the most earnest work that you have ever done in your life, to resolve that this is going to be the greatest, the most courageous and the most sinless year of life that you have ever lived; I want you to make up your minds to do this; to decide that you are going to continually grow.... There are but two directions in this life in which you can grow; backward or forward. You can grow stronger, or you can grow weaker; you can grow greater, or smaller; but it will be impossible for you to stand still.

NOVEMBER 27

Practice Gratitude for Stories

Self-Care, Identity

I had written as far as this when Piglet looked up and
said in his squeaky voice, "What about *Me*?"

"My dear Piglet," I said, "the whole book is about you."

. . . And now all the others are saying, "What about
Us?" So perhaps the best thing to do is to stop writing
Introductions and get on with the book.

A. A. MILNE, *Winnie-the-Pooh*

Throughout the course of your life, stories have shaped you: the tales
about dreamers and adventurers that delighted you as a child, the stories you heard from friends about their life experiences, the comedies
and dramas you've seen played out in films.

Take a few minutes to create a list of stories that have been the most
meaningful to you. These could be from friends, in books, in films, or even
in song lyrics. How have these stories shaped your dreams, desires, and
calls to action?

NOVEMBER 28
Watch Figure Skaters Train
Experience

The ice for miles together had been swept clean by the
wind, and was like a vast, glaring sheet of plate-glass.
Most of it was a deep, brilliant green. Here and there
would be stretches of milky ice, and now and then great
rounded patches would suddenly meet them, which were
black or deep brown.

ERNEST INGERSOLL, *The Ice Queen*

Indulge your childhood self and head to an ice-skating rink to watch
figure skaters practice their routines. As thrilling as it is to watch the
best of the best compete in the Olympics, there is a certain magic to
watching skaters in the building process—honing their skills and per-
fecting their grace. Imagine how many falls it took for the elite athletes
to reach their optimum skill level.

It's easy to idealize and celebrate the star athletes or the top achiev-
ers in any area, but the real victories take place day in, day out, with
each fall that leads to another try.

NOVEMBER 29
Everything Counts
Whimsy

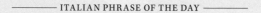

———— ITALIAN PHRASE OF THE DAY ————

Tutto fa brodo: everything makes broth, soup

This Italian expression means every little thing counts. Every ingredient added to your life contributes to the whole—even small pinches of spices can help make exquisite soup.

Apply this Italian mindset to your own life. Whether it be saving five dollars a week for that special item you've been eyeing, spending ten minutes of time on a passion project, or simply sharing a smile and greeting as you walk through your neighborhood—it all adds up and makes a difference.

NOVEMBER 30

Imagine All the Dreams Your Heart Desires

Dream

The future belongs to those who believe in the
beauty of their dreams.

ELEANOR ROOSEVELT (ATTRIBUTED)

This time of year invites us to examine our lives with gratitude and to
cultivate appreciation for the blessings in our everyday. As we regard
the present with joy, let us also offer thanks for the dreams we keep in
our hearts—the quietly held hopes and whispered wishes that we hold
dear when we look toward the future. Take some time to imagine the
fulfillment of your wide-eyed aspirations, and delight in imagining the
dreams your heart desires.

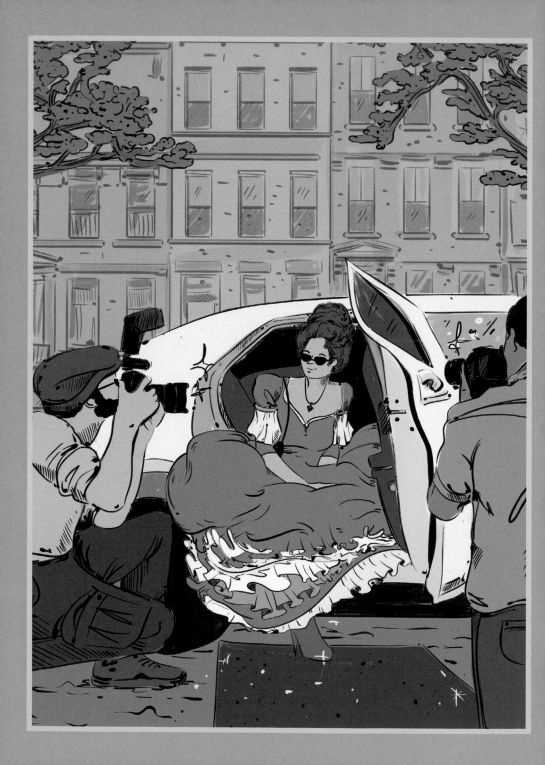

December

DECEMBER 1
List of Comforts
Coziness

Make a list of the things that bring you the most comfort and make you feel the most at peace and grounded. Intentionally incorporate at least one of those things into every day this month.

DECEMBER 2
Find Your Winter Scent
Beauty, Identity

Welcome the winter with your signature scent for this season! Let the spices of autumn carry into these colder months, with notes of cinnamon, nutmeg, and gingerbread, and lean fully into winter, with scents like frosty peppermint, rich pine, or sophisticated cedarwood and sage.

DECEMBER 3
Be the Leading Lady
Identity, Self-Care

In the movies we have leading ladies and we have the best friend. You, I can tell, are a leading lady, but for some reason you are behaving like the best friend.

NANCY MEYERS, *The Holiday*

It's sometimes easy to get so wrapped up in supporting the lives and dreams of those around us that we lose sight of our own desires. Where does this leading-lady mentality need to shine through in your own life? If you aren't quite sure, carry this thought with you, and see where it chooses to emerge throughout this week.

DECEMBER 4
Bake Up Some Holiday Cheer
Connect

Bake holiday cookies to give to friends or neighbors! Whip up some old favorites along with some new recipes. And don't skimp on the sprinkles.

DECEMBER 5
Watch for Magic
Whimsy, Dream

Above all, watch with glittering eyes the whole world around you because the greatest secrets are always hidden in the most unlikely places. Those who don't believe in magic will never find it.

ROALD DAHL, *The Minpins*

DECEMBER 6
Deck the Halls
Home, Create

Decorate your home for the holidays! Hang sparkly lights, make cheerful garlands, put up seasonal knickknacks. There's no rule book here—just indulge in whatever sparks joy for you, and the result will be magical.

DECEMBER 7
Choose Your December Theme Song
Whimsy

Imagine this year as a slideshow of snapped photographs: the momentous occasions and the fleeting feelings, the celebratory days and the cozy, quiet nights. Choose a song that honors every one of them.

DECEMBER 8
Winter Affirmations
Self-Care, Identity

What good words do you need to hear this winter? With the approaching holiday season, you may be spending lots of time and energy thinking about how you can take care of those around you with food, gifts, and quality time spent together. Take a little time to think about how you can care for yourself as well by writing down your winter affirmations. When you take good care of your own emotional needs, you'll be better able to take care of those around you.

DECEMBER 9

Reflect on Admiration

Connect

Reflect on a quality you admired in a person whom you interacted with today. What was the scenario that highlighted the quality you admire? How did it feel to witness it? How did that character trait affect others? Keep your eyes open tomorrow for another quality you admire. You'll be amazed by the sense of gratitude and awe this practice cultivates in you to view your interactions through this seeking perspective.

DECEMBER 10

Donate to a Family in Need

Experience

The holiday season can be especially stressful for families with financial strain. Look into how you can support families in need through community centers, homeless shelters, faith-based organizations, or hospitals.

DECEMBER 11
Host Your Own Cooking Show
Create, Connect, Whimsy

Tonight you are the star of the show! As you prepare dinner, narrate each step as if you were on a cooking show. Explain the chops, note the measurements, comment on the flavors, and try your best not to burn anything. Maybe even enlist a friend to do the same. Then you can trade videos and teach each other some of your favorite go-to recipes in a way that's so much more fun than sending a list of ingredients.

DECEMBER 12
Make a Winter Wreath
Create, Nature

Bring the outside in by making a winter wreath. Head to a local garden nursery and see if they have any greenery scraps available to take for free. (They often do around the holidays.) Then purchase any additional greenery, branches, or blooms you want to add to your wreath.

Look up tutorials on how to weave and layer the branches and stems together to create a beautiful wreath. Hang it on your front door or any location that could use some added cheer!

DECEMBER 13
Write Your Own Remix
Experience, Create

Stretch yourself outside your comfort zone and exercise those creative muscles by writing your own remix. Take a song you know well (preferably with a catchy beat), pick a topic you want to write about, and dive in!

DECEMBER 14
HELLO, LOVER
Javaphile
Whimsy

Javaphile: a person who loves to drink coffee

There are coffee drinkers and then there are *coffee lovers*. These are the café dwellers, the ones who grind their own beans, and then there are some who even source beans from independent growers and roast their own.

If you're a javaphile like so many others, branch out and try a new café, a new roast, or a new coffee drink today.

DECEMBER 15

RECALIBRATE YOUR MORNING ROUTINE

Carve Out Quiet Time

Self-Care

Create a sacred space for quiet time each morning. Whether you spend this time praying, meditating, reading, or simply just being, it is hugely beneficial for helping you approach the day with a sense of calm and peacefulness. Resist the temptation to pick up your phone and scroll through the news, social media, or your email inbox. Allow yourself the gift of lingering in the dreamy coziness of these precious early-morning moments.

DECEMBER 16

Gingerbread Home-a-Rama

Connect, Create

Host a gingerbread house–making contest with all the festive candy fixings. Decide on awards ahead of time! A few ideas are: Most Likely to Be Featured in a Snow Globe, Most Creative Design, Best Use of Candy Decorations, and Most Delectable-Looking.

DECEMBER 17
Go on a Twinkle-Light Adventure
Whimsy, Experience, Connect

Invite a friend or two to take a drive or walk with you to look at holiday lights. Look up "most festive holiday houses" in your area if you want to see the most decked-out locales. Make warm drinks to bring with you, turn on festive music, and enjoy the sights!

DECEMBER 18
Start Your Own Holiday Tradition
Whimsy

One of the fun parts of being an adult is that you get to call the shots for your life, and that includes the traditions you choose to practice. This season, create a new holiday tradition that is meaningful for you. It could include friends and family or it could be a solo venture. Reflect on what thoughts, feelings, values, and experiences you want to cultivate during the holidays, and start a tradition of your own!

DECEMBER 19
You Are Beautiful!
Create, Connect

A high-school student named Shea Glover conducted a social experiment where she photographed people, then captured a second photograph after she told them they're beautiful, and their expressions are priceless.[26] Try telling someone they're beautiful today and watch their face light up! And don't forget to look in the mirror and tell yourself.

DECEMBER 20
Wrap a Gift with Grandeur
Create

Invest some extra time and effort to wrap a gift with grandeur, creating an experience for the loved one who will receive the offering. You could tie up the package with multiple styles of ribbon, use a unique wrapping paper—or even newspaper for a creative and classic touch! Give special attention to the name tag, or add a snip of greenery to the top. Opening the gift may become just as exciting as the gift itself.

DECEMBER 21
Take What You Need
Whimsy, Self-Care

Take what you need, and carry it with you for the rest of your day:

- delight in the celebrations of this season
- excitement for the year ahead
- gratitude for the goodness that came from the past year
- acceptance of the coexistence of highs and lows

DECEMBER 22
Visit a Greenhouse
Experience, Nature

Colder temperatures and fewer hours of daylight have likely kept you inside more during the past few months. If you're not too caught up in holiday festivities, you may notice your soul craving the doses of nature you enjoyed this spring, summer, and fall. If so, a warm, vibrant oasis might just be within your reach.

Check out a local greenhouse, where you'll find respite from winter's cold amid the warm air, diverse flora, and abundant foliage.

DECEMBER 23
Make a Double Batch
Connect, Create

Gather enough ingredients to make two times the amount of food you need for this evening's dinner. Enjoy the first half of the batch, and drop off the second half of the meal for a friend who is feeling stretched a bit thin these days.

DECEMBER 24
Make a Floral Arrangement
Create

Head to the store and buy a variety of winter blooms, greenery, and dried plants for a beautiful floral arrangement. Look up inspiration pictures, or just follow your intuition! Above all, enjoy the process of piecing together these beautiful blooms to create your own floral masterpiece.

DECEMBER 25
Reflect on Gifts
Self-Care, Identity

Gifts come in all shapes and sizes, from relationships and experiences to impactful words and objects we use every day. Today reflect on your life's gifts and your gratitude for them.

Take a few moments to journal about some of the best gifts you've received in your lifetime: the gifts you hoped and prayed for, the gifts you never thought you'd receive, the gifts that caught you by surprise and gave you exactly what you didn't know you needed.

DECEMBER 26
Go to the Zoo
Experience, Nature

While a trip to the zoo may not be top of mind during the colder months, many zoos put up elaborate light displays this time of year. Enjoy a winter walk surrounded by exotic animals and twinkle lights!

DECEMBER 27

HELLO, LOVER

Astrophile

Whimsy

Astrophile: a person who loves stars or astronomy

When was the last time you looked up at the stars? Can you identify the Big Dipper and Little Dipper? Try using a sky map or star chart to identify some of the major stars and constellations and fall in love with the night sky.

DECEMBER 28

Step Up Your Bath Game

Self-Care, Home, Coziness

Plan a luxurious bath night. Prep the little indulgences that will create your personal oasis. This may include Epsom salt, relaxing essential oils, a face mask, flickering candles, a speaker to hum the perfect background music, or a tray to hold a book or beverage.

Draw the bath, set the mood, and hop in! Take a few moments to unwind—it's your night! Remember, there is no right or wrong way to enjoy this time.

DECEMBER 29
Honor Your Elders
Connect

This time of year can be especially tough for those who feel alone. So many men and women in nursing homes don't have family or friends who come to visit them. Call a nursing home in your area to see if they have any residents who could use some company, and stop in for a visit. Bring a deck of cards or a few books that you can offer to read aloud. Most importantly: be present, ask questions, and offer a willing ear to listen. This small act of kindness will do as much for you as it does for the person with whom you spend this time.

DECEMBER 30
Live the Full Life of the Mind
Whimsy

Live the full life of the mind, exhilarated by new ideas, intoxicated by the Romance of the unusual.

ERNEST HEMINGWAY, *The Complete Short Stories of Ernest Hemingway*

DECEMBER 31

Appreciate the Extraordinary Miracles of This Year

Self-Care

> What is it you plan to do with your one wild and precious life?
>
> MARY OLIVER, "The Summer Day"

Today marks the end of another year and the beginning of a new one.

Spend some time reflecting on the extraordinary miracle that you are alive, right here and right now. Take a deep breath, and revel in the beauty of this present moment. Appreciate the past that led you here; look forward to the days ahead with hope.

This life of yours is filled with beauty and wonder, sorrow and celebration, seasons of challenge and change, and peaceful moments of knowing you're exactly where you're meant to be.

You, friend, have been given the gift of life.

What will you do with it?

Notes

1. "Remembering Julia Child in Her Centenary Year," Le Cordon Bleu, https://www
   .cordonbleu.edu/news/julia-child-centenary-year/en.
2. "8 Greek Words for Love That Will Make Your Heart Soar," Dictionary.com,
   February 2, 2022, https://www.dictionary.com/e/greek-words-for-love/.
3. Eric Suni, "Circadian Rhythm," Sleep Foundation, updated January 18, 2023,
   https://www.sleepfoundation.org/circadian-rhythm.
4. Rebecca Joy Stanborough, "A Hobby for All Seasons: 7 Science-Backed Benefits
   of Indoor Plants," Healthline, September 18, 2020, https://www.healthline.com
   /health/healthy-home-guide/benefits-of-indoor-plants.
5. Rebecca Seiferle, "Romanticism Movement Overview and Analysis,"
   TheArtStory.org, September 25, 2017,https://www.theartstory.org/movement
   /romanticism/.
6. Ornish Living, "The Science Behind Why Naming Our Feelings Makes Us
   Happier," *Healthy Living* (blog), *HuffPost*, updated December 6, 2017,
   https://www.huffpost.com/entry/the-science-behind-why-na_b_7174164.
7. Jennifer Larson, "What Is the Purpose of Theta Brain Waves?" Healthline,
   July 1, 2020, https://www.healthline.com/health/theta-waves.
8. "Floriography: The Secret Language of Flowers in the Victorian Era," *Planterra
   Conservatory* (blog), https://planterraevents.com/blog/floriography-secret
   -language-flowers-victorian-era.
9. "Transcript: Michelle Obama's Convention Speech," NPR, September 4, 2012,
   https://www.npr.org/2012/09/04/160578836/transcript-michelle-obamas
   -convention-speech.
10. Marianna Pogosyan, "In Helping Others, You Help Yourself: The Benefits of
    Social Regulation of Emotion," *Psychology Today*, May 30, 2018, https://
    www.psychologytoday.com/us/blog/between-cultures/201805/in-helping
    -others-you-help-yourself.
11. Alain De Botton, *The Art of Travel* (New York: Penguin Random House, 2002).
12. Annette McDermott, "6 Ways Your Body Benefits from Lemon Water,"
    Healthline, updated May 6, 2022, https://www.healthline.com/health/food
    -nutrition/benefits-of-lemon-water.

13. Mayo Clinic Staff, "Honey," Mayo Clinic, https://www.mayoclinic.org/drugs
    -supplements-honey/art-20363819.
14. "Florence Nightingale," History.com, November 9, 2009, https://www.history
    .com/topics/womens-history/florence-nightingale-1.
15. Edgar Munhall, "Elsie de Wolfe," *Architectural Digest*, December 31, 1999,
    https://www.architecturaldigest.com/story/dewolfe-article-012000.
16. Jennifer Stone, "How to Calculate How Much Water You Should Drink,"
    University of Missouri System, https://www.umsystem.edu/totalrewards
    /wellness/how-to-calculate-how-much-water-you-should-drink.
17. "The History of Fountains," *Water Gallery* (blog), February 21, 2018, https://
    www.watergallery.net/blog/the-history-of-fountains/.
18. "What Does Ikigai Mean in Japanese?" Ikigai Living, accessed January 30, 2023,
    ikigai-living.com.
19. Erin Eatough, "What Is Ikigai and How Can It Change My Life," *BetterUp* (blog),
    May 7, 2021, https://www.betterup.com/blog/what-is-ikigai.
20. Robert N. Kraft, "10 Benefits of Making Lists: Understanding the Allure of List-
    Making," *Psychology Today*, May 7, 2021, https://www.psychologytoday.com/us
    /blog/defining-memories/202105/10-benefits-making-lists.
21. Katherine Kam, "Self-Awareness Can Improve Relationships. Here Are
    Tips to Build It," *The Washington Post*, November 26, 2022, https://
    www.washingtonpost.com/wellness/2022/11/26/self-awareness-emotional
    -intelligence/.
22. "Diwali: Festival of Lights," *National Geographic Kids*, accessed December 9, 2022,
    https://kids.nationalgeographic.com/pages/article/diwali.
23. Liz Schumer, "What Is Diwali? The History Behind the Important Holiday,"
    Good Housekeeping, October 29, 2021, https://www.goodhousekeeping.com
    /holidays/a37680263/what-is-diwali-history-story-celebration-facts/.
24. Sunny Fitzgerald, "The Secret to Mindful Travel? A Walk in the Woods,"
    National Geographic, October 18, 2019, https://www.nationalgeographic.com
    /travel/article/forest-bathing-nature-walk-health.
25. "Mother Teresa," Biography.com, April 2, 2014, https://www.biography.com
    /religious-figure/mother-teresa.
26. "Wonderful Social Experiment Shows People's Reactions to Being Told They're
    Beautiful," Digital Synopsis, accessed December 9, 2022, https://digitalsynopsis
    .com/inspiration/people-react-to-being-called-beautiful/.